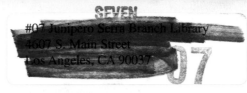

KNACK®
MAKE IT EASY

DIABETES COOKBOOK

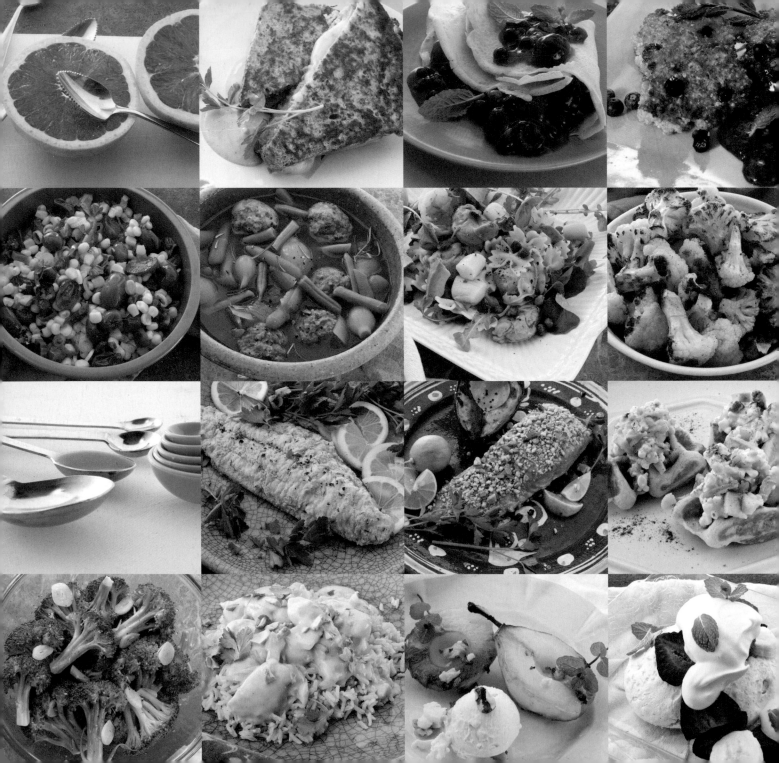

KNACK®

DIABETES COOKBOOK

A Step-by-Step Guide to Delicious, Healthy Meals

NANCY MAAR

Technical Review by Nancy Held, M.S., R.D., C.D.E.
Nutritional Information by Jean Kostak, M.S., R.D., C.D.E.

Photographs by Viktor Budnik

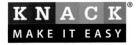

Guilford, Connecticut
An imprint of The Globe Pequot Press

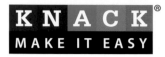

Copyright © 2009 by Morris Book Publishing, LLC

Editor in Chief: Maureen Graney
Editor: Katie Benoit
Cover Design: Paul Beatrice, Bret Kerr
Text Design: Paul Beatrice
Layout: Maggie Peterson
Cover photos by Viktor Budnik
Edited by Linda Beaulieu

All interior photos by Viktor Budnik with the exception of p. 18 (left): © Gsermek Dreamstime.com; p. 18 (right): Kerry Garvey/ Shutterstock; p. 19 (left): Shutterstock; p. 19 (right): © Vladmax Dreamstime.com; p. 29 (left): © Alamy; p. 34 (left): © Monkey business Dreamstime.com; p. 34 (right): © Dreamstime.com; p. 35 (left): © Josefbosak Dreamstime.com; p. 35 (right): © Jjphotos Dreamstime.com; p. 93 (right): © Ever Dreamstime.com; p. 97 (left): © Rorydaniel Dreamstime.com

Library of Congress Cataloging-in-Publication Data is available on file.

ISBN 978-1-59921-506-8

The following manufacturers/names appearing in Knack Diabetes Cookbook are trademarks:
Colman's
Corningware
CrockPot
Cuisinart
Earth Balance
Kashi
Pyrex
Rival
Splenda
Tabasco
Wondra

Printed in China

10 9 8 7 6 5 4 3 2 1

Dedication

To my mother, Patricia, a diabetic with a sweet tooth and a sweet nature to match

Photographer Acknowledgments

I would like to say thanks to all at Knack. Thanks to my crew of gifted and talented people—Claire Stancer, a wonderful and talented food stylist who created beautiful food to shoot, and JCH, a great prep/assistant and food shopper for this book.

—Victor Budnik

CONTENTS

INTRODUCTION

Healthy Cooking: An Introduction

Healthy cooking is not about depriving yourself of the foods you love, but rather about adopting a health-conscious lifestyle that allows you to cook the foods you love and crave, but with fresh, healthier ingredients and a greater understanding of your fundamental nutritional needs. Healthy cooking is a lifestyle decision, and one that can be made with relative ease by following some of the quick tips provided throughout this book, including buying fresh foods locally, occasionally using salt and sugar substitutes, and being mindful of what you are eating.

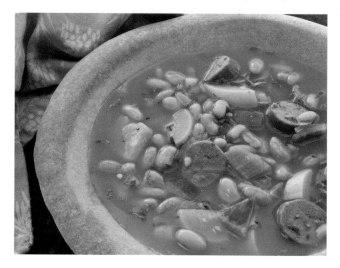

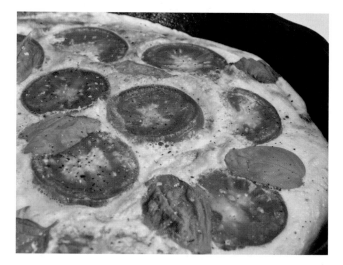

The *Knack Diabetes Cookbook* provides you with healthy, balanced, mouth-watering recipes for every meal of the day, whether it's savory stuffed French toast for breakfast, a warm lentil salad for lunch, or a Mediterranean rice and seafood casserole for a hearty dinner. Being healthy does not mean compromising on taste; in fact, by using fresh ingredients, taste is often enhanced.

For someone with diabetes, the most important thing to consider is downsizing portions. You can eat a wide variety of foods and still maintain good blood sugar control by eating lots of fresh fruit and vegetables, whole grains, and lean meat, fish, and poultry. "All in moderation" is a good motto to follow when planning out your meals for the week.

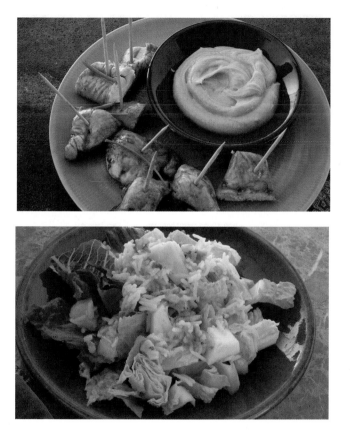
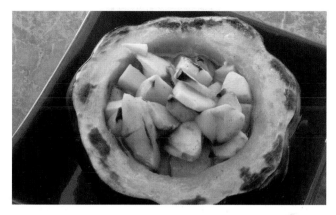
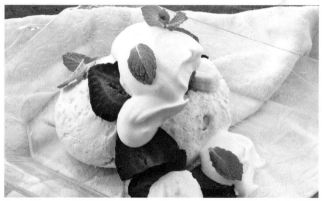

This cookbook also helps you stock your kitchen and your pantry, providing information on the essential equipment and food items needed to create a balanced, delicious meal for you and the ones you love. Included are wonderful recipes for homemade ketchup, mustard, vinaigrettes, and other dressings and sauces, which are perfect for finishing touches on a grilled vegetable salad or a pistachio-pepper strip steak.

In a short time, you'll find you can indulge your cravings and feed your family—and yourself—healthy meals that are good for both the soul and the body. So please flip through these pages and get inspired.

Healthy Eating: A Diabetes Educator's Perspective

What does healthy eating mean for someone with diabetes? It is essentially the same as for one without diabetes but with attention to specific issues. Healthy eating is the first priority for people with diabetes. This means a diet with high-quality carbohydrates and fiber, low in saturated fat, and calorically appropriate to attain weight loss or maintain weight. Controlling carbohydrate intake and monitoring blood sugar can go a long way toward achieving glucose control.

Carbohydrate is the nutrient that affects blood sugar the most compared to other dietary components. Foods that

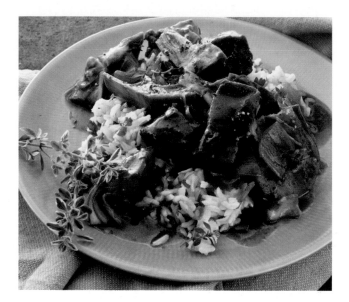

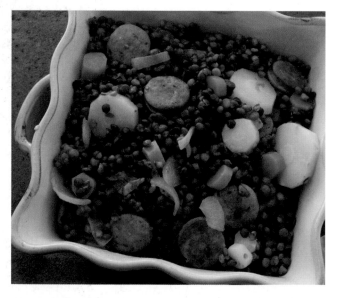

contain carbohydrates are potatoes, bread, cereals, pasta, and starchy vegetables such as peas and corn. Milk, yogurt, and fruit also have carbs. Vegetables have carbohydrates but in small amounts. Fiber is a carbohydrate but affects the blood sugar less than starch and sugar. Monitoring blood sugars with a home blood glucose meter is critical to effective diabetes self-management. Observing how food, activity, and other factors affect blood sugar assists in making changes.

Carbohydrate counting is a helpful tool in controlling blood sugar and can also help reduce caloric intake. In basic carb counting, one learns how much carb is in foods and the amount to eat at meals and snack. Those on rapid-acting insulin can adjust the insulin depending on the amount of carb eaten. Another method to control food intake is the American Diabetes Association (ADA) Food Exchange system. This tool organizes food according to nutrient content.

People with diabetes may be given guidelines by their diabetes educator based on carb counting or the exchange system. For those who count carbs, I suggest that 30 to 60 grams of carb may be in a meal and 15 to 30 grams of carbs in a snack. Of course, the grams in each meal depend on the overall amount in the meal plan and caloric level desired.

The glycemic index (GI) is a ranking of foods based on their effect on blood sugar levels. It is a measure of how fast carbohydrate-containing foods raise the blood sugar. There are many factors that affect the GI, but generally foods that are less processed and have more fiber, such as vegetables,

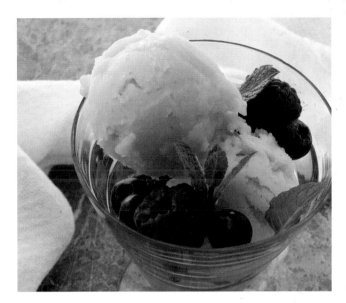

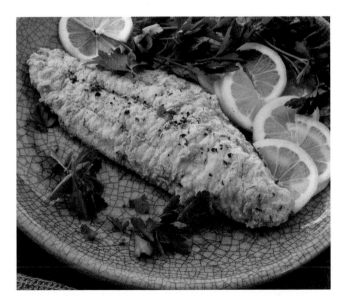

fruits, beans, whole grains, cereals, and breads, produce a slower blood sugar rise.

Since heart disease is one of the potential complications of diabetes, dietary factors that impact on cardiovascular disease should be modified. Saturated and trans fats have the most adverse effect on blood fat levels. These include animal fats, e.g., butter, sour cream, high-fat meats, and whole-milk dairy products. The fats to choose are omega-3 fats (salmon, really any fish has some of this healthy fat, walnuts, flax) and monounsaturated fat (olive and canola oil, avocado, nuts, olives).

The key to successful diabetes control is learning how to self-manage—paying attention to blood sugar, making reasonable changes in food or lifestyle, and eating healthfully to prevent or minimize diabetes complications.

—Nancy Held, M.S., R.D., C.D.E.

FOODS FOR HEALTHY LIVING
Essential foods include fruit, vegetables, proteins, and olive oil

Every kitchen should be stocked with a supply of healthy food: fruit, vegetables, proteins, olive oil, and whole grains. It should exclude "bad carbs" and fats. Bad carbs contain processed sugars and bleached flour. Butter, cream, whole milk, and ice cream should be substituted with olive oil, nonfat milk, and sugar-free sorbet.

The fruit in your diet may include any fresh, frozen, dried, or canned fruit. If canned, it must be packed in water, not syrup. Vegetables include dried grains and legumes as well as green and yellow varieties. Green and yellow veggies may be fresh, frozen, or canned. Proteins include cheese, meat, fish, eggs, dairy, and legumes. Olive oil works well with vegetables. In addition, the human body needs some healthy carbs. Good carbs are less processed ones, such as

Fresh, Dried, and Canned Fruit

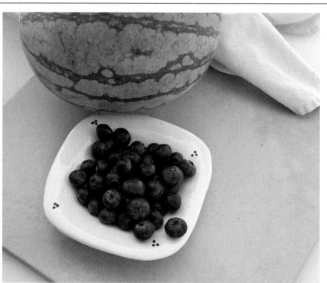

- Fresh fruit is the best to use in recipes and, when locally grown, will have spent the least amount of time in a refrigerator or on a train or truck.

- Be exceptionally careful of canned fruits – even packed in light syrup, they'll be loaded with cane sugar syrup.

- Some frozen fruits are also packed in sugar.

- Dried fruits concentrate the natural sugars. However, the fiber helps to overcome the sugar content.

Vegetables and Grains

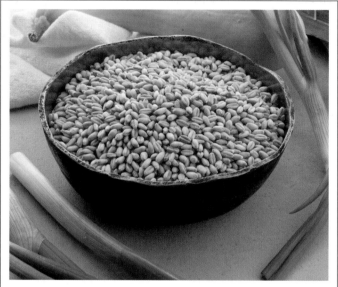

- Be careful of white, processed flour in breads and cereals. Always look for whole-grain breads, pastas, and cereals.

- Yellow vegetables are important. Carrots, yellow summer squashes, and parsnips are good examples.

- Tubers, including potatoes, and root vegetables such as beets, parsnips, and carrots, though sweet, are part of a healthy diet.

- Fill up on low-cal, "good carb" spinach, broccoli, and cabbage for health.

whole grains, fibrous fruits, and vegetables.

A healthy kitchen should also limit fats and not so healthy carbs. The carbs to avoid are the white ones, including processed flour, white sugar, and any products made with them. Fat should be minimized in most cases, since they are so calorically dense. Even though certain oils actually heighten your good cholesterol, all fats and oils contain the same amount of calories. For example, one tablespoon of butter contains the same number of calories as one tablespoon of oil.

········· GREEN ● LIGHT ·········

Depending on where you live, you will find fresh food at green markets and roadside stands all year round. If you live in a northern region, it's a good idea to freeze as much of the fresh summer fruits as possible to use in winter recipes. A peach pie in February, made from fruit that you've blanched, cut up, and packed with lemon juice, can literally bring summer to the table even though the snow may be flying outside.

Protein

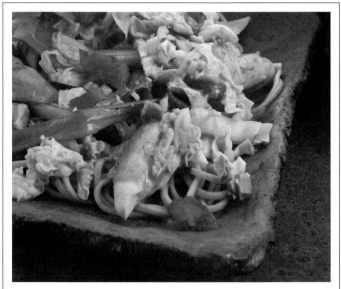

- Protein is a building block of strength and health. There are many forms of protein, from vegetable sources, such as legumes, to low-fat milk, yogurt, and cheeses.

- Lean meats, such as chicken, turkey, veal, and lamb, are good sources of protein. Just be sure to cut off all of the fat from the meat before cooking.

- Fish is an excellent source of lean protein.

- Some grains, such as quinoa, have a significant amount of protein.

Oil

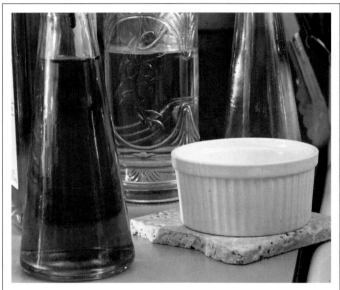

- When you must use fat, choose olive oil, canola oil, and the oils from peanuts and various vegetables.

- Hydrogenated oils should be avoided. They stick to the arteries like glue.

- The process of hydrogenation makes oils solidify, so these oils will look and act more like butter, a saturated fat.

- Fats and oils from animals are very bad for arteries. Fried foods should be avoided, as should fatty meats, such as bacon, ham, sausage, and some cold cuts.

STOCKING YOUR PANTRY

Have your favorite basics stored conveniently, and keep them well-organized to ease and expedite food preparation

The pantry can be a small- to medium-size room, a cupboard, or a closet; all you need to have are shelves to store food. Shelves along the basement stairwell or in a dry basement will also serve as a pantry.

Items that are not perishable are kept in the pantry. Sugar and flour need to be put in airtight containers to prevent

them from attracting bugs or getting moldy if it's damp.

Dry items, such as pasta and rice in airtight containers, canned goods, and items in bottles all go into the pantry. Cookie and apothecary jars and tins in various sizes will hold cookies, rice, beans, and flour.

Assemble all of your baking supplies in one area. Include

Baking Supplies

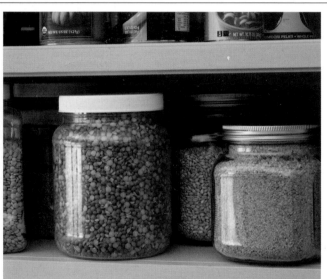

- Shelf organization is handy for keeping everything you need for one kitchen task together. If there is room to keep baking pans, pie pans, cookie sheets, and muffin tins together, then do so.

- Keep flour, sugar, salt, baking soda, and powder in neatly labeled contain-

ers. Keep bottles of vanilla extract and other flavorings on hand, too.

- Keep your extra cake and biscuit mixes (if you use them) in the pantry.

- Rice, pasta, and soup mixes should all be stored in the pantry area.

Spices

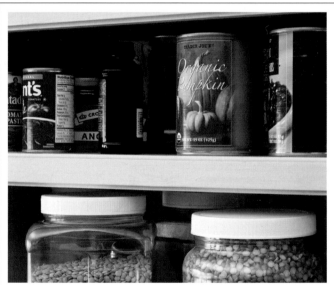

- Keep the flavorings and spices that go with your baking supplies right with them. These include vanilla and almond extract, cinnamon, nutmeg, whole cloves, and ground cloves.

- Honey, maple syrup, and salt substitute should be stored here, as well.

- Keep your canned nuts with the baking supplies.

containers of flour, sugar, baking powder, large boxes of salt or salt substitute, and bottles of vanilla.

Put your dry pastas in another area, with your canned tomatoes and tomato paste. Condiments that do not need refrigeration can also be stored in the pantry. Bottles of ketchup, Worcestershire sauce, hot sauce, etc., can be stored here.

Herbs should be closer to the workspace, typically next to the stove. Cans of ground coffee, jars of instant coffee, and tea, can be stored on shelves in airtight containers, such as jars.

MAKE IT EASY

If you live in an apartment with little cupboard space, you have to scale down your supplies. Get stackable glass or plastic holders for bulky items. Glass is excellent for storing items because you can see what's in it. Label each container. To expand space, add shelves to rooms with high ceilings, cupboards, and closets. Hanging wire baskets also serve as storage for onions, potatoes, fruit, and veggies.

Canned Goods

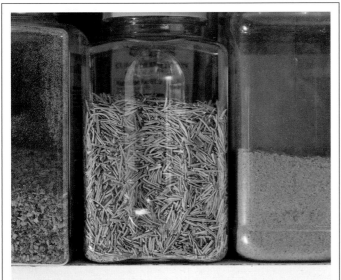

- Place all of your dried fruits and nuts in airtight containers or resealable plastic bags.

- Keep your canned fruits and fruit juices together, arranging the smaller sizes at the front and the tall ones at the back.

- Keep any canned vegetables together.

- Broth in cans and dried legumes for soup-making can all be put together.

Extra Containers

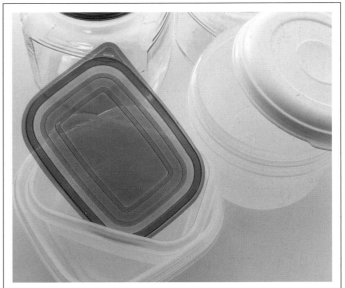

- It's important to have plenty of plastic containers of various sizes on hand.

- You will also need tins for open packages of cookies and crackers.

- Mason jars are good for holding open boxes of tea, coffee, etc.

THE REFRIGERATOR
Use this space wisely to store all of your perishables

Before electric refrigerators were invented, people had wooden ice boxes. Ice was delivered by horse-drawn cart daily during the summer and every few days in winter. Housekeepers would put a sign for ice in the window, and the man with the cart would deliver it to the kitchen door. This was true of homes and apartments.

Thankfully, refrigerators came right along with electricity and were common by the 1920s. What a blessing! With refrigerators, food stays fresher longer. When stocking your fridge, remember that local foods bought daily are freshest.

A well-organized fridge is key for any cook; it allows for items to be found more quickly and minimizes the chances that foods will go bad while sitting hidden in the back of the fridge. Foods should be organized with like foods (veggies

Foods That Last One Day

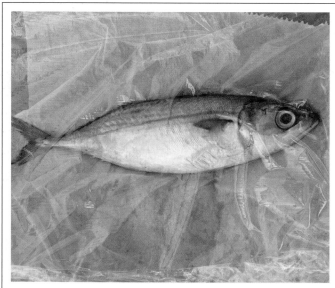

- Fresh fish (buy it the same day or the day before you plan to use it). Fresh or defrosted shrimp, scallops, crab, and lobster meat.

- Completely defrosted ground meat and chicken.

- Freshly picked, ripe berries and cut up fruit (these will last overnight).

Foods That Last up to One Week

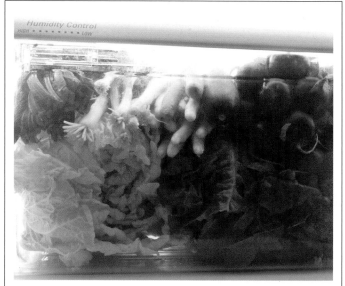

- The way veggies are packaged dictates their fridge life. Some plastic bags keep soft vegetables fresh for up to one week.

- Fruits and veggies that have been in the refrigerator for too long get limp, moldy, or gooey at the edges.

- Homemade soups and stews are good for one week. Soft fruit lasts one week if not ripe.

- All foods should be labeled with the date you packaged them. Push older things to the front, and, if possible, add to soups or stews as soon as you can.

with veggies in crisper drawers, for example) and, if opened, should be labeled with expiration dates. Be sure to check these expiration dates regularly to ensure that you're using fresh foods. Foods that have passed their expiration date can make you and your family sick if they are eaten.

Keeping a running grocery list will also ensure that you never run out of a key ingredient right when you need it most. When you discover that you're running low on a certain item, add it to your list for the next time you go grocery shopping.

· · · · · · GREEN ● LIGHT · · · · · · · ·

Keep your fridge clean: Wash it out every two to three months with a solution of dishwasher detergent, white vinegar, and 1 teaspoon of baking soda to deodorize it. Remove the veggie drawer; wash it thoroughly to clean away any mold. If there is mold in your refrigerator, you breathe the spores every time you open the door. If mold gets into your sinuses or lungs, it can make you very sick. Even a small refrigerator can harbor dangerous mold.

Foods That Last for One Month

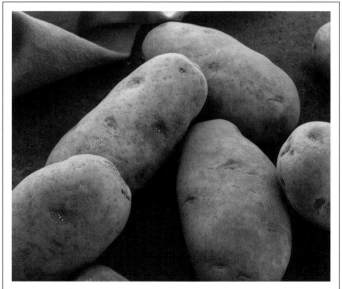

- Foods that last for one month include unopened vegetables, soups, broth, and other well-packed and well-sealed items.

- Always look at the "sell-by" dates on any packaged foods you buy that you plan to keep for a while.

- If you buy onions in a plastic bag, take them out of the bag; these bags are often moist inside and will contribute to spoilage.

- Always check your refrigerator for "science projects" – things that were pushed to the back and forgotten.

Keep Track of Foods

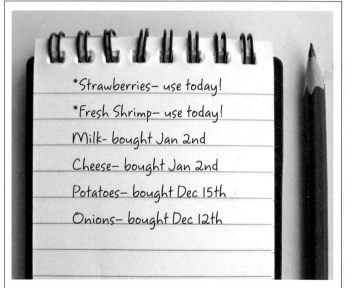

- List foods as you buy them.

- Star foods to be used right away.

- Cross off foods as you use them to add to next shopping list.

- Plan meals in advance to use up ingredients already in your refrigerator.

THE FREEZER
The freezer might be the greatest food storage tool since canning

Freezers are a great place to store foods that you intend to use long-term. Frozen items do not last forever; however, if you use a vacuum packer to freeze them, you'll find that they do last months longer than if you simply wrap them in plastic. The vacuum packer is especially good for individual servings of meats, fish, etc.

Liquids, such as soups and stews, frozen fruits, and tomatoes, should be stored in plastic containers with tight tops. Chicken, beef, and vegetable broth are available for soups, stews, and sauces when frozen in two-cup to quart containers.

Freeze items such as peeled and grated fresh ginger by the tablespoonful in small bags. Lime and/or lemon juice can be frozen in ice cube trays and then placed in plastic bags.

As with your refrigerator, be sure to organize like food items

Freezing Herbs

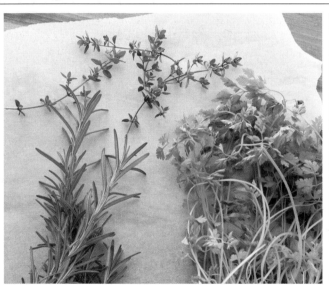

- To freeze fresh herbs, first rinse and dry them.

- When they are dry, prepare a cookie sheet with parchment paper.

- Lay the herbs on the parchment paper and place in the freezer for 1 hour.

- Label plastic bags with names of the herbs you are freezing. Place the herbs in plastic bags and keep frozen.

Freezing Berries

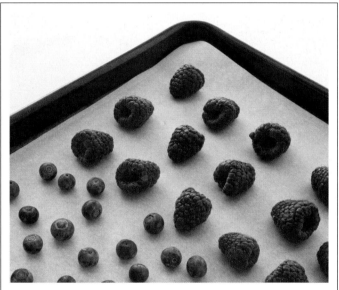

- Wash and dry ripe berries, leaving them whole; remove stems after washing or the juice will run out.

- Place a piece of parchment paper or aluminum foil on a cookie sheet.

- Spread the berries on the sheet so they are not touching. Place in the freezer for at least one hour and no more than three.

- Place the berries in plastic bags and return to the freezer for future use.

together so that they're easy to pull out and use. Also, label all food with their expiration dates so that you know the latest date when you can to use them.

There's nothing less appetizing than a piece of meat or fish that's been in the freezer for too long. Freezer burn is a drying out process that makes it too late to use the item as intended. In the case of steak or a roast, you might cut it into stew meat.

GREEN ● LIGHT

Freezer Night: Every two to three months, it's a good idea to go through your freezer and make a surprise dinner. Even if the freezer items don't seem to go well together, you may find yourself with a smorgasbord of delights. By doing this, stored food doesn't have a chance to become freezer burned or otherwise tired. Combine leftover chicken soup and veal stew to make a pot pie, for example.

Freezing Tomatoes

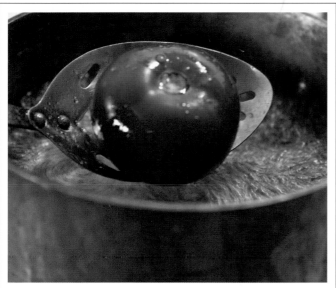

- Freeze tomatoes for soup, sauces, or stews.

- Bring a pot of water to boil. Put a few tomatoes at a time into the water. Place a colander in your sink.

- Blanch tomatoes by adding them to the boiling water a few at a time. Boil three to four minutes, until skins are loosened. Place the tomatoes in the colander.

- Let them cool, then pull off skins. Cut tomatoes in quarters and place in plastic containers with about 1 teaspoon lemon juice as preservative. Cool before freezing.

Freezing Peaches

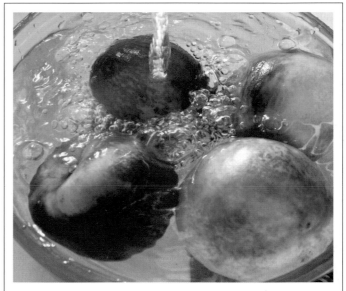

- Ensure that you'll have fresh pies, tarts, and flan all winter.

- Bring a pot of water to a boil. Place a few peaches at a time in the boiling water. Boil three to four minutes. Place a colander in the sink.

- When skins loosen, place peaches in the colander to drain and cool. When cool enough to handle, slip skins off and cut fruit in halves, removing the pits.

- Place halved peaches into a freezer container. Sprinkle each layer of fruit with fresh lemon juice. Cover; freeze.

FRESH FOODS

Chefs and good cooks agree, the fresher the food, the better

Fresh foods are always a good option when cooking up a delicious meal. Fresh foods often taste more vibrant than frozen options, and many are often grown locally, which supports the community.

Proper storage of fresh foods in your kitchen is paramount for ensuring the quality of the food. Place items you want to ripen, such as avocados and melons, in a sunny window. If you want these items to ripen slowly, place them in a cool, dark area of your pantry or in the refrigerator. Most fresh foods are refrigerated. Even "winter" vegetables keep longer when refrigerated. Salad greens are the most delicate. Cabbage, escarole, chicory, kale, spinach, mustard greens, and collards should never be left out at room temperature.

When buying veggies from the market, remember to dry

Using Fresh Fruit

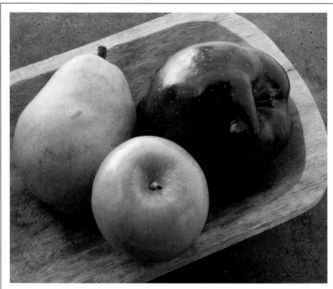

- Pears, apples, and bananas do not have to be refrigerated if they are going to be used promptly. If you have a cool pantry, place pears, apples, and bananas there.

- Always wash fruit before eating or cooking it to remove any pesticides or germs.

- Don't wash fruit until just before you are ready to eat it. The moisture will hasten the rotting process.

Colorful, Nutritious Dinners

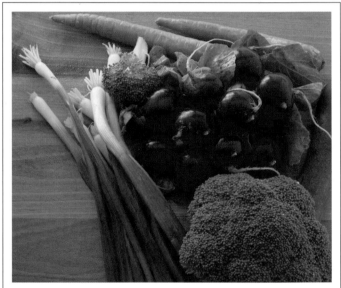

- Use as much color as you can find in the produce section of your market. Get greens (lettuce), reds (tomatoes), and yellows (peppers, carrots) into your meals.

- Peppers are excellent garnishes, while baby spinach goes happily into soups, stews, and omelets.

- Buy sale greens in the supermarket or at the farmstand, or use what's flourishing in your garden. Go seasonal for fresh. Always look for the darker greens, as they have more nutrition.

- You can also buy frozen vegetables. Nutrition quality is not lost in freezing.

them before storing. Most supermarkets "mist" their vegetables. This makes them glisten and look appealing, but the moisture rots the vegetables very quickly. Always dry fruit and especially salad greens before storing. Use a salad spinner or a kitchen towel.

Always smell fish and seafood before buying. Make sure fish has shiny scales and bright eyes. Fresh seafood and fish will keep for only a short amount of time in your fridge, so be sure to make a note of expiration dates and use those ingredients within a few days.

Add Greenery to Salads

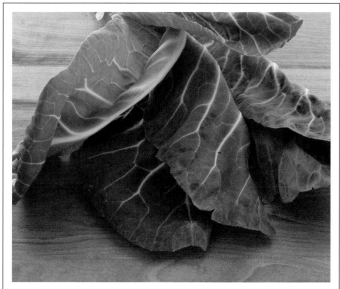

- When making salads, add darker greens to iceberg lettuce or Napa cabbage. Greens come in all sizes, from small and bitter, such as arugula and watercress, to large and sweet, like romaine and iceberg lettuce.

- Before using heads of lettuce, remove outside leaves. Slice lengthwise and then crosswise. Add shredded watercress or arugula for extra nutrition.

- For good measure, rinse greens at this point. Wrap all greens in paper towels before storing in plastic bags.

Preparing Fresh, Aromatic Vegetables

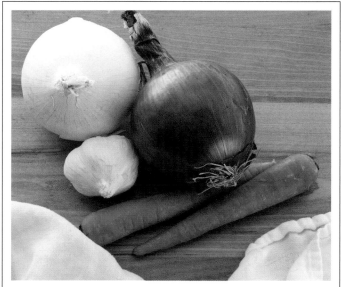

- Aromatic vegetables include carrots, parsnips, celery, onions, garlic, and turnips. They add flavor, fiber, and minerals to your recipe repertoire.

- Prepare garlic by breaking it into cloves. Slam cloves with the side of a cleaver, which separates them and makes them easy to peel. Place in a plastic bag in the fridge for quick access, or slice and freeze.

- Cut off and discard ends of onions; peel and chop. Place in freezer. Peel and slice carrots and parsnips; store in the fridge. Potatoes should be peeled at the last minute.

FLAVORINGS

Every kitchen should have a variety of flavorings, from oils and vinegars to herbs, spices, and extracts

When thinking about the kinds of flavorings to add to your recipes, start with the basics: salt substitute or sea salt, black peppercorns and red pepper flakes, or ground red pepper (cayenne) and pepper sauce.

You will also need herbs. All herbs begin as green leaves. You may grow your own or buy herbs fresh, dry them yourself, or buy dried herbs in bottles. Basic herbs include basil, oregano (the darling of the pizza parlor), thyme (think of turkey stuffing), dill weed for fish and seafood, and sage for all sorts of soups and stews. There are hundreds of others.

Spices include twigs, roots (such as ginger), seeds (mustard, fennel, anise, coriander, celery seed, and dill seed), and

Acidic Dressings

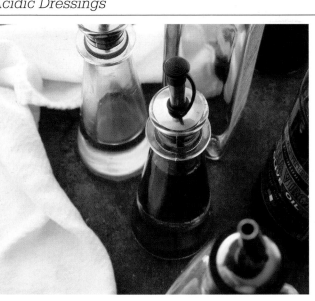

- Every salad needs an acid for flavoring, to counterbalance oil and bring out the flavors of greens.

- Basic dressing is made of one part vinegar and three parts oil. Vinegar can be flavored by red or white wine, sherry, raspberry extract, and various herbs, such as

basil and tarragon. Lemon or lime juice can be added or substitute for vinegar.

- Orange juice is a nice cooking liquid.

- Mixed dressings are blends of mayonnaise and citrus or vinegar. These include green goddess and Caesar.

Oils

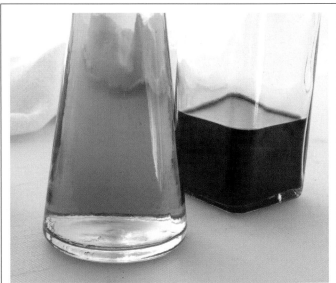

- Oil is a crucial ingredient in almost all dressings, marinades, soups, stews, and sauces. Extra virgin oil comes from the first pressing. Virgin olive oil (the second pressing) and plain olive oil (the third) are often mixed with other oils.

- Once you've added vinegar,

spices, and herbs, only an educated palate can tell the difference between pure olive oil and blends.

- Salads, broiled or sautéed chicken, duck, fruit, or seafood will be dry without oil in some form, whether it's olive, canola, peanut, flavored, or mayonnaise.

dried berries (cumin, pepper, juniper berries, nutmeg, cloves, and allspice).

Other important flavors come from extracts, such as vanilla, lemon, and almond. Sauces, such as soy, Tabasco, and Worcestershire, are combinations of spices and a carrier. Many flavored oils are also useful in the kitchen. Oils include the basics, canola and olive oil, as well as sesame seed, walnut oil, and truffle oil, for starters.

Wines also make excellent flavorings. Red and white wines that are good enough to drink are good in small amounts.

Sherry and Marsala have strong flavors and should also be used sparingly.

A well-stocked kitchen will have the basic flavorings ready and available. When stocking your kitchen each week, remember to check your herbs, spices, and extracts for any necessary refills. Chances are, you'll be using these ingredients a lot in your dishes.

Bottled Flavorings

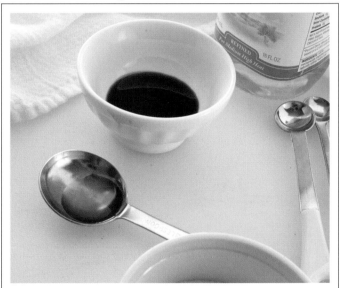

- When setting up your kitchen, you'll find that there are many goodies to add to the above-mentioned oils, vinegars, and spices.

- Worcestershire sauce and low-sodium soy sauce are invaluable as soup and stew flavorings. They don't require refrigeration and can be used in lieu of steak sauce on grilled meats.

- Always refrigerate opened barbecue sauces, ketchup, and chili sauce; pickles, roasted peppers, and artichokes; olives, ground coffee, and mayo. Don't refrigerate extracts or unopened jams or jellies.

Sugar Substitutes

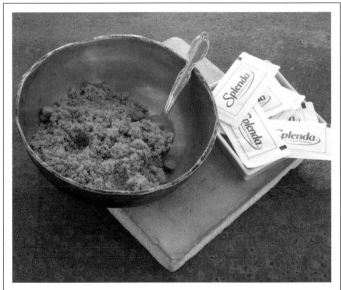

- Store your sugar and sugar substitutes in airtight containers. They absorb humidity and the steam from boiling, broiling, and poaching.

- Brown sugar substitute is important to baking, and in chili sauce and barbecue sauce.

- White sugar substitutes labeled "for baking" have some real sugar in them.

- But without the real sugar, the baked product will be dry, with a coarse texture.

SMALL TOOLS

These kitchen implements are key for preparing delicious and nutritious recipes

There are four small tools that you should always have on hand in your kitchen: a lemon/lime reamer, a wire whisk, a box grater, and a small spatula. Many of the recipes in this book use fresh lemon or lime juice. Lemon/lime reamers are generally wooden and fluted to twist out the juice and pulp.

Wire whisks come in many sizes, from tiny to huge. A medium-size whisk is useful for beating eggs, whipping cream, whipping egg whites, and generally mixing things up.

A box grater is essential if you don't have a food processor. And for many recipes, the box grater works just as well. Use it for cheese, carrots, etc.

A small turner or spatula is also essential. Not just for turning

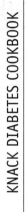
A Lemon Reamer

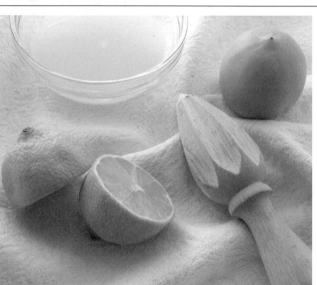

- With a lemon reamer, you can control quantities of liquid, from a few drops to half the lemon (or lime).

- Lemon juice is essential to flavor fish and prevent fruit from discoloring.

- It also keeps the colors true in vegetables. Lemon juice is used in sauces, braises, and dressings.

- Lemon wedges are used as garnishes, and lemon "cures" foods, cooking the food in its acidity.

A Wire Whisk

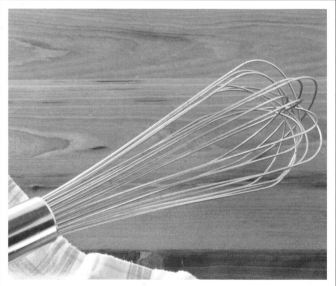

- The wire whisk is useful for beating eggs. It's also fine for whisking egg whites into a mass of peaks and for whipping cream.

- The whisk is also useful for getting lumps out of sauces.

- When making pan gravy, use the whisk to break up

- the brown bits on the bottom of the pan while adding hot liquid. This requires a good whisk.

- The whisk is also good for making salad dressings, blending the oil and acid thoroughly.

food as you cook it, but for peeking under pancakes and such to check for doneness.

Some other small tools are also great to have on hand: A garlic press pushes a peeled clove of garlic through a small, heavy fine sieve. The smaller the garlic is cut, the stronger. For making garlic bread, the garlic press produces very small bits that are liquid. This is also a good way to add garlic in salad dressings. A tiny citrus stripper to remove thin strips of lemon, lime or orange peel is excellent for adding twists, and making garnishes for many dishes. Keep it with your lemon reamer. A mandolin is handy for making paper-thin slices of cheese, onions, potatoes, or other vegetables. Be careful to get the type of mandolin with a holder. If you have to hold the food while you move it across the blade, you may easily slice the tips of your fingers.

The Box Grater

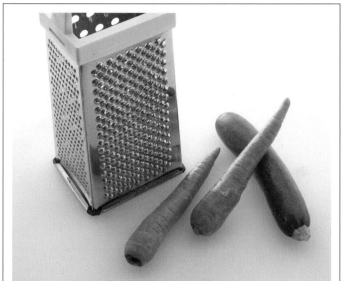

- Box graters may be old-fashioned, but they are extremely useful. Each side has a function. One wide side grates; the other wide side slices; one small side scrapes and the other is a minigrater.

- Grating is done on one side. It is easier to control than a food processor.

- Scraping is done on the other side of the box. Use the rasp to zest a lemon or lime quickly.

- The slicing side is fine for various types of vegetables, such as cucumbers.

A Plastic Spatula

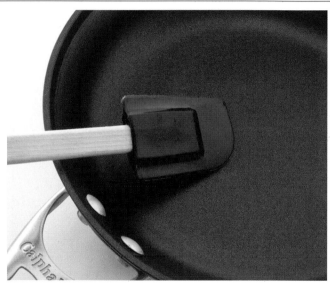

- A small spatula is useful for turning your crepes and omelets.

- It's also good for checking under an omelet to see if it's browning nicely.

- A small spatula can be used for scraping up brown bits on the bottom of a pan.

- Plastic spatulas are more versatile than metal ones, as metal spatulas cannot be used in nonstick pans.

SMALL, SHARP CUTTING TOOLS

Cooks need easy access to knives, peelers, kitchen shears, and grapefruit spoons

When it comes to cutting and prepping food, a seasoned chef will turn time and again to certain kitchen essentials. A set of really good, sharp knives, from a short paring knife to a serrated bread knife to a cleaver, is important because cooks need different knives to cut, slice, and chop. Dull knives are dangerous, as they slip off the food and into fingers. Many

good knives are sold in sets with a knife sharpener, which is a worthwhile investment.

A really good knife is worth the gold you spend for it. Cheap knives do not sharpen properly. They will tear, even bruise the food rather than cutting through it. English and German steel knives are excellent. Old-fashioned carbon steel knives

A Knife Set

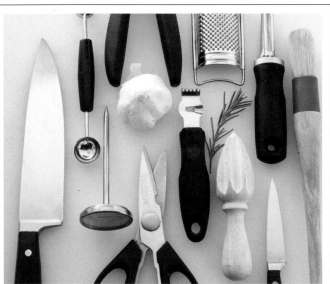

- A knife set has knives for various purposes. A paring knife is used to cut the hulls from strawberries, pare off the skins of small vegetables, and remove stems.

- A serrated knife is for bread and slicing cakes. It acts like a saw and does not crush the bread or cake.

- A chef's knife, with its slightly curved blade, is excellent for carving meat and poultry.

- A cleaver is important for chopping, dicing, and mincing vegetables and other foods.

Vegetable Peelers

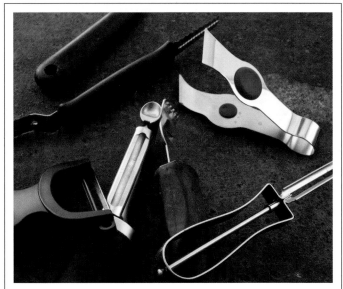

- When you find a style of vegetable peeler you are comfortable with, buy a couple. Throw out dull ones; if you are preparing a big meal, get others to help peel.

- Peeling techniques vary, and for left-handed cooks, the crossbow style is best

- for agility. Get the sharpest stainless-steel peeler you can find.

- Adjust your stroke speed and length depending on the food you peel. Some work best with small strokes, while bigger foods, such as full-size eggplants, work well with long strokes.

aren't pretty, as they turn dark gray and can rust, but they are easily sharpened to a razor's edge.

Peelers come in two designs, the "crossbow" and the "up and down." Either works well if the peeler is sharp. Use peelers for vegetables and tubers. Every kitchen needs scissors, both heavy shears for cutting up a chicken, and smaller ones for opening plastic bags, cutting string, etc.

Perhaps the most surprising tool necessity here is the grapefruit spoon, which has a pointed tip good for removing grapefruit and orange sections and many other uses.

MAKE IT EASY

Honing your knife: Knives must be kept sharp with either a honing stone or a flint "pencil" on a wooden handle. Simply hone your knife with a few strokes on each side every time you use it, always moving in the same direction. Then, store the knife so that it isn't rattling against other knives and utensils, which could chip or otherwise mar the blade. Serrated knives and steak knives do not need to be sharpened.

Kitchen Shears

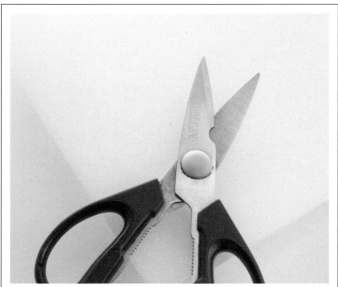

- Shears are essential for a variety of jobs. Little jobs include cutting string and opening plastic packages.

- Big jobs include cutting up a chicken and cutting various parts of meat, which is easier to do this way and more accurate than sawing away with a knife.

- Large kitchen shears are excellent for cutting the wing tips from turkeys, ducks, and chickens for the stockpot.

- You also may find them more convenient and easier to wield than a knife for cutting up baby back ribs.

The Grapefruit Spoon

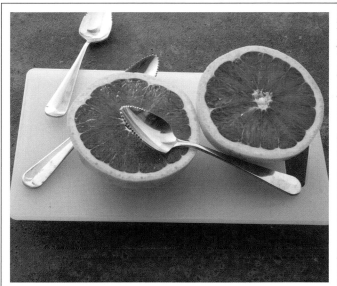

- The grapefruit spoon is as delicate as a surgical tool when used with a little practice and skill.

- It was originally designed for segmenting grapefruit for eating. Its genius is in the spoon's slender tip. This works around pits, seeds, and skins.

- When making baked potato skins, cut the raw potato in half and scoop out the pulp with the grapefruit spoon.

- Use the spoon to scoop out avocados, melons, and the cores from apples and pears.

MEASURING TOOLS

Measuring tools come in handy when baking, while weight tools work wonders for entree recipes

When you are adding broth to your stew, a ½ cup more or less doesn't make much difference. When you are baking a cake, however, an ounce more or less of flour, baking powder, or sugar can mean success or failure.

There are two kinds of measuring cups: dry and liquid. The liquid measures are almost always glass, so you can see the quantities glazed on the sides of the cups. These are available in 1-, 2-, and 4-cup sizes. Dry measuring cups are individual, from ¼ cup to 1 cup. They are generally plastic or stainless steel, nested, and tied together. Many measuring cups have both grams and ounces printed on the sides.

Measuring spoons from ⅛ teaspoon to 1 tablespoon work

Dry Measuring Cups

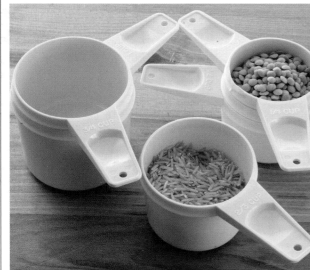

- When you are measuring flour or sugar with dry measuring cups, overfill the cup.

- Then, take a knife and level off the top so that it's perfectly even.

- If the recipe calls for the flour to be sifted, use a

sifter or a sieve, then return it to the measuring cup. You'll find that fluffed up by sifting, there's more volume.

- Be sure to use the knife again to scrape off the extra flour.

Liquid Measuring Cups

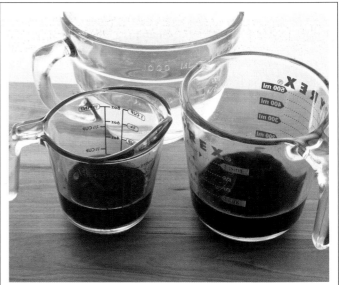

- When cooking, you need to know the quantities of the liquid measurements.

- Two cups equal one pint; four cups equal one quart.

- Grams, cubic centimeters, and liters are different, and here's where the numbers

on the other side of the measuring cups work, when you are using a European recipe or following a diet that's measured in grams rather than in ounces.

- You can make close approximations of a recipe in grams and liters.

for dry and liquid measures. For people on theraputic diets, these are small and accurate scales for measuring food.

There is one caveat: Although measuring spoons are based on using teaspoons and tablespoons, it is best not to use them for measuring. This is because the bowls of the spoons are shallower than those of measuring spoons. You are more likely to spill your vanilla extract when using a teaspoon from your flatware set than with a measuring spoon. Also, with a set of measuring spoons, the ½ teaspoon and ¼ teaspoon sizes are included, too. An ⅛ teaspoon is equal to a pinch or a dash.

It's best to use measuring cups; a teacup is not really eight ounces; it's more like five or six, depending on the set. And coffee mugs run the gamut from six to ten ounces. So especially when baking but even as a general cooking rule, use dry and liquid measuring cups to be exact.

Measuring Spoons

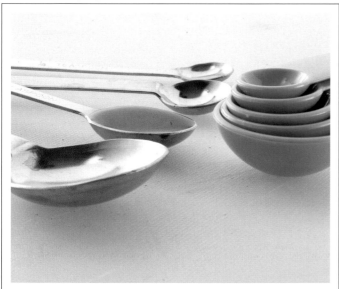

- Plastic measuring spoons are kept together by a plastic ring. The metal spoons are kept nested by a metal ring.

- Many cooks detach them for easy use; if you use but one while it's still attached, you end up having to clean them all.

- If you detach them, it's easy to misplace parts of the set. So detach and then store them in a ziplock bag.

- Measuring spoons will give you a more accurate measurement than your flatware spoons due to the depth of the spoon.

Old-Time Measuring

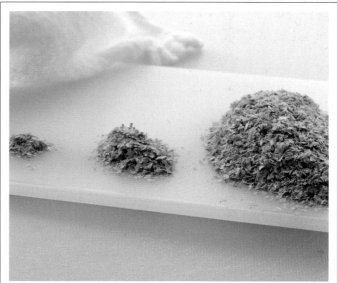

- If you come across an old family cookbook and want to translate, here's a guide:

- The old silver or stainless teaspoon or tablespoon is equivalent to the measuring spoon.

- A pinch is equal to ⅛ teaspoonful. A dash is equivalent to a ½ teaspoon.

- A handful is equal to about four ounces or a half cup.

LESS USED BUT NECESSARY TOOLS

While you may not use these items on a daily basis, always keep your kitchen stocked with them

Many of the gadgets you see in the gourmet cooking stores are not absolutely necessary, but they are fun. When looking for kitchen gadgets, think about the foods you like to eat every day. Are you big on salad or spinach? In that case, you will probably need both a colander and a salad spinner in your kitchen. Sieves and colanders are necessary for rinsing

fruit and vegetables. You can also use the salad spinner as a colander for large, leafy vegetables.

If you rarely blanch and freeze tomatoes yourself, on the other hand, you probably don't need a food mill, since a traditional food processor works fine for occasional use. Some gadgets can be used for multiple purposes. Fine sieves, for

Sieves and Colanders

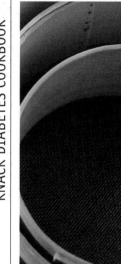

- Aside from rinsing and cleaning food, a fine sieve can be used for making a puree. By pushing berries or tomatoes through, seeds and lumps are removed.

- If you do not bake often, use a fine sieve in place of a sifter.

- A large colander is excellent for washing spinach and lettuce. It's easy to put the colander in a large pot of cold water and swish lettuce around to remove the dirt.

- When you remove the colander from the water, you should have clean leaves.

Salad Spinners

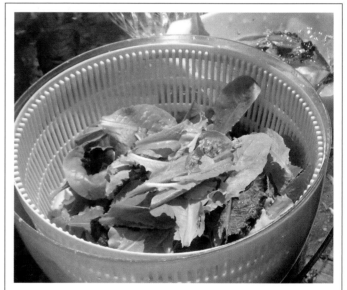

- These clever inventions use centrifugal force to spin water off the leaves.

- After you wash your greens, spin them as dry as possible. Drain off the water in the bottom of the container and spin the greens again for good measure.

- If you are storing the greens, wrap them in paper towels and then place them in a plastic bag.

- Greens will stay crisp in the refrigerator for four days.

example, are used to separate out small foods, but they can double as sifters. You'll find that sifters are most important for baking. Depending on your needs, you will determine what is necessary and what isn't. Many chefs will agree, however, that the following tools, while perhaps not used often, are still a great addition to your gadget collection.

When organizing your kitchen, remember to keep these tools tucked away in an easy-to-reach location for occasional use.

MAKE IT EASY

If you run out of shelf space to store you gadgets, try this: Use pegboard with holes in it for hooks to hang your gadgets. Arrange your least-used mills, colanders, and sieves where they are out of the way. Use a tea tray with a shelf or a bread rack with vertical shelves for storing small appliances. Also check out your local container store or hardware store for various other forms of accessible storage.

Sifters

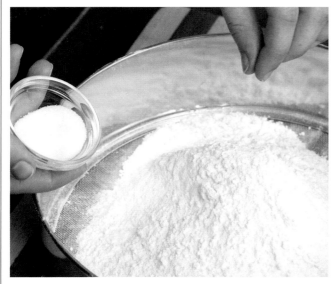

- Cooks who do a lot of baking need sifters. Since most recipes call for two to three cups of flour, a three-cup sifter is about all a home baker needs.

- Sifting is more important when making cakes than it is when making pies.

- After the flour is sifted, it must be returned to the dry measuring cup for readjustment.

Food Mills

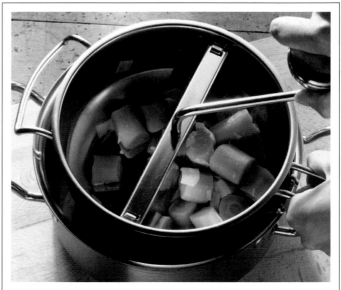

- Food mills are available in both electric and hand-crank models. They have been in use by cooks for years.

- Food mills separate the skin and seeds from the pulp of tomatoes and berries.

- Mills can be found in very large sizes for cooks who are canning large amounts of tomatoes or for cooks who make jams and jellies.

- Mills preceded the food processor, which purees food but does not remove the seeds, instead simply grinding them up with the skins.

SMALL APPLIANCES

These gadgets are important and handy to have around the kitchen

While not every appliance is needed for a gourmet kitchen, every kitchen does need a food processor, a blender, and two electric mixers, one hand-held for small jobs and a large, standup one for making whipped egg whites (for use in soufflés, for example).

Food processors are equipped with blades that have different uses. The basic grinding blade also chops, minces, and purees. It works well with carrots, onions, and nuts. It is an alternative to a blender for pureeing soups and smoothing out sauce. The grating blade works from the top down, while the basic blade works from the base up. It grates potatoes, carrots, cabbage vegetables, and cheese, among other things. The slicing blade works well on vegetables, such as carrots and cucumbers, for salad. It also slices potatoes very

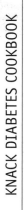

Immersion Blender

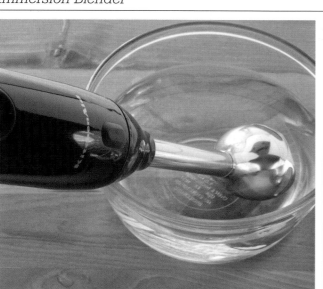

- Immersion blenders are good for mixing foods together, especially smoothies and sauces.

- There are some disadvantages, however; some hand-held blenders can slop food or liquids over the side of the bowl. Some are difficult to clean. It is best to experi-

ment with various sized bowls and varying levels of liquids, starting with water.

- To clean, immerse the blender in hot, soapy water. Turn on the motor and run it until the blades are clean. Rinse the blender under hot running water first, then immerse it in cold water.

Food Processor Blades

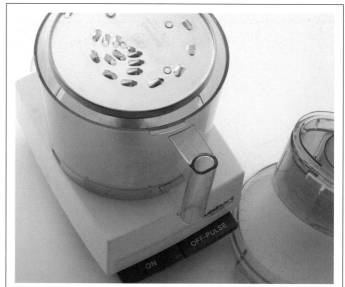

- The food processor blades chop, mince, and puree, but not as finely as does the blender. Use this gadget to chop onions and garlic for soups or to chop veggies for stews.

- The grinding blade chops when you pulse it. You

can fine- or coarse-chop nuts, veggies, and fruits by starting and stopping, i.e., pulsing your processor. The longer the machine is on, the finer the chop will be. Use the slicing blade for thin slices of celery or cucumber, or for the potato pancake recipe.

efficiently. The food processor can do most of what a blender does, but blenders are not as versatile as food processors.

Blenders are, however, important, especially for making smoothies, fruit sauces, and salad dressings. Some blenders are equipped with a mini jar, which is great for making small quantities of salad dressing.

Hand-held and standup electric mixers are useful for beating eggs and making flan batter, cake batter and small omelets.

Hand-Held Electric Mixer

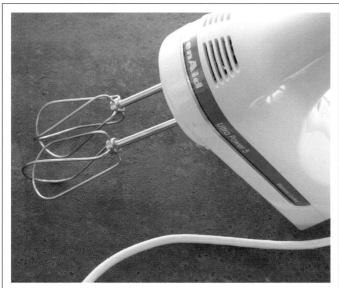

- The hand-held electric mixer can be used for a variety of things. Use it to mash potatoes for a very good consistency.

- The hand-held electric mixer also works well for beating eggs for the World-Class Scrambled Eggs recipe.

- Use this mixer to beat eggs for omelets. The Egg White Omelet recipe will be puffier if you use the mixer to whip up the whites.

- You can also use the mixer for a variety of baking needs.

Standup Electric Mixer

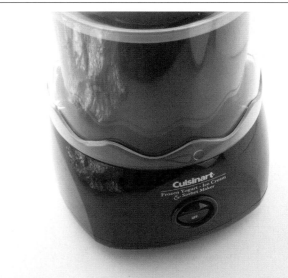

- Many electric mixers have a whisk attachment as well as kneading blades for use in making dough that requires kneading.

- The standup electric mixer is most useful when you are cooking for a crowd and making dishes by the quart rather than in small quantities.

- The standup electric mixer also frees you up to do something else while the mixer does the work.

MID-SIZE APPLIANCES

These kitchen items will help expedite many dishes and save you time in the kitchen

Every chef can appreciate the help of some time-saving appliances in his or her arsenal of tricks. The microwave, toaster oven, and slow cooker are three items a modern-day chef should not live without. Even a luxury item like the ice cream/sorbet maker will help make things easier for the gourmet chef.

A microwave helps with faster prep times. When you have green beans, asparagus, or brussels sprouts, you can preheat them in the microwave, ready in ninety seconds. Carrots, parsnips, and winter squash soften up quickly in the microwave.

A toaster oven is great for snacks, such as crostini. You can also use it for fast top-browned, toasted sandwiches, melting cheese on omelets, and fast-toasting nuts. An ice cream/

Microwave

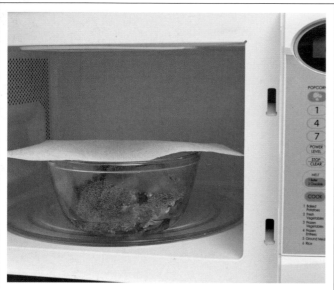

- Of the myriad things you can do with a microwave, cooking veggies is prime.

- Try this: Trim an artichoke; cut off bottom and outside leaves. Put artichoke in a glass bowl with 2 tablespoons of water and 1 teaspoon of lemon juice. It will be ready in four minutes.

- Always cover food with freezer paper, waxed paper, or paper towels.

- Never cover food with plastic wrap, as plastic releases harmful chemicals, considered carcinogens, that leach into your food.

Toaster Oven

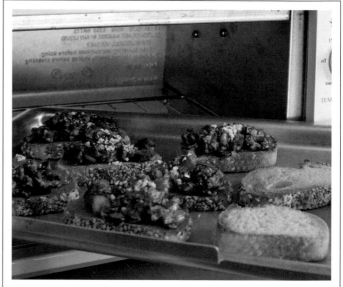

- Use your toaster oven for baking small quantities, for browning, and, of course, for toasting.

- Handy and easy to use, from warming a batch of brownies to heating and toasting some garlic bread, toaster ovens are great appliances.

- When you have several people at breakfast, most toaster ovens will hold four split English muffins at one time.

- Bran muffins and bagels do not do well in the microwave. However, you can toast several of them at a time in the toaster oven.

sorbet maker is excellent for controlling the sugar in your desserts, a big help for people with strict dietary needs.

Slow cookers are a household favorite, with different varieties, sizes, and brands available. Slow cookers make dinners easy for the working chef, who sometimes may not always have the most time in the world to prepare a five-star meal. Slow cookers make it easy: Make your broth or stock and simmer your hearty soups and stews.

Ice Cream Maker

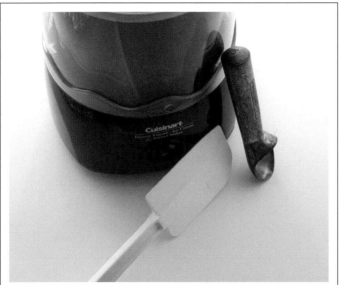

- When using an ice cream maker, be sure to follow the directions exactly and never overfill your ice cream freezer.

- If you do, the appliance will overflow as the ice cream churns.

- Make sure that all of your ingredients are very cold before adding them.

- Set aside toppings such as more fruit, nuts, and raisins to eat with the ice cream, sorbet, sherbet, or frozen yogurt.

Slow Cooker

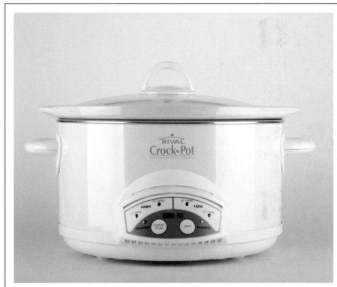

- Slow cookers are made from heavy ceramic ware. These thick pots are excellent heat carriers.

- Aside from soups and stews, there are plenty of recipes that are easy and good in the slow cooker.

- Make your pot roasts in the slow cooker, for example.

- Keep an eye on your slow cooker the first time or two that you use it so that you will know if it over- or under-heats.

SAUTÉING

The sauté technique is used for vegetables, meats, and fish

The art of sautéing is a versatile skill that every good cook should learn. A sauté pan is made of tin or stainless-steel–lined copper, heavy stainless steel, enamel-clad metal or good-quality nonstick material. The sauté pan is not as deep as the frying pan. It can be substituted for a wok when stir-frying but is not as conveniently designed for moving food from hot to warm.

Aromatic vegetables are sautéed prior to using them in soups, stews, and braises. Meats such as filet mignon and veal scallopini are also sautéed or pan-fried, keeping it low fat. The same is true of delicately fleshed fish, such as fillet of sole or flounder.

Even when you use a nonstick pan, it's wise to add a bit of olive oil or nonstick spray. The first part of the sauté is to

Preparing to Sauté

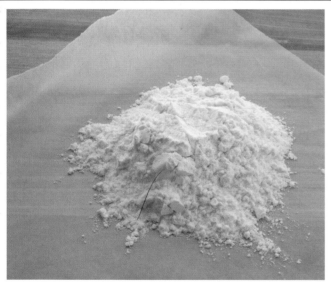

- First, sprinkle a piece of waxed paper with flour, salt, and pepper. You can add herbs at this point.

- Thoroughly dry the piece of meat or fish you plan to sauté. Do this to avoid making a gooey mess when you dip it in flour.

- Heat the pan over medium-high heat. Add the oil or nonstick spray to the pan.

- Start to brown the food.

Wait for the Sizzle

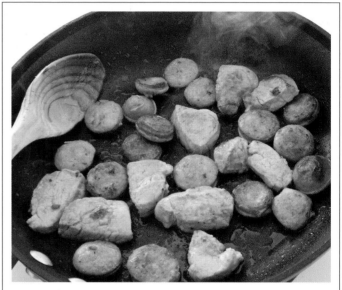

- Listen for the sizzle before lifting the food for a peek. When the meat or fish starts to sizzle, look under it with your turner or spatula.

- When you see that it's nicely golden on one side, turn the meat or fish.

- At this point, you probably will want to turn the heat down.

- Cooking time depends upon the thickness of the meat or fish.

sear the food. This means putting it on a very hot pan. This seals in the juices and gives it nice color. It's also called caramelization, as heat browns the food, bringing out the juices, starches, and sugars. You need only enough olive or canola oil to coat the bottom of the pan.

Butter should not be used since it has a low burning-point and will not get as hot when cooked. Whereas, grapeseed oil can get hot without burning. The searing part of a sauté is enhanced by adding a dusting of flour to food. It forms an attractive crust when you do not want to use high heat.

Pan-frying

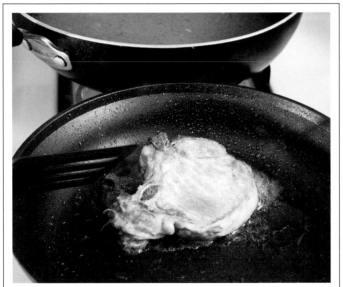

- It is quick to sauté thick pieces of meat on top of the stove. When you sauté (pan-fry) meat, it means less clean up.

- First, as with thin cuts, sear the meat on a medium-high to high flame. After you've turned it, reduce the heat to low.

- Cover the pan and let the filet mignon or chop cook for three minutes. Turn and cook for another three minutes for medium rare.

- Give it four minutes more per side for well done. Always rest the meat in a warm place, covered for at least five minutes.

Using Sauté Drippings

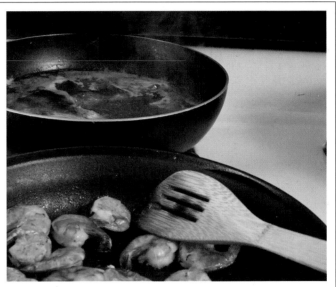

- Once you've finished sautéing, you'll see brown bits in the bottom of the pan.

- These are nuggets of flavor and the base for a sauce.

- If you've cooked chicken, add ½ cup of chicken broth; if beef, the same; if a lamb or veal chop, add chicken broth. With fish, add water or clam broth.

- Raise the heat to medium and simmer, stirring. Add ¼ cup of red wine for beef or ¼ cup of white wine for fish or chicken. Season with pepper and your favorite herbs.

BRAISING
This technique is a progression from sear and sauté to simmer

Braising is an age-old technique. It sears in the juices and then adds liquids and flavors for a long, slow simmer on top of the stove, in the oven, or in the slow cooker. Braising produces warming comfort food, the stuff of cold winter nights and chilly days out-of-doors.

Chili, stew, fricassee, and pot roast are all braised. When you make chili, the liquids become gravy and carry the flavors of the dish. Everything is blended into a wonderful marriage. With stew, the pieces of meat retain some of their individuality. A pot roast is mostly meat with enough gravy and vegetables to be delicious and moist. A chicken fricassee is made of pieces of chicken that have been browned, and then vegetables and lots of cornstarch gravy are incorporated.

Remember, too much heat at the wrong time makes food

Equipment for Braising

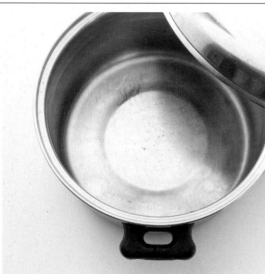

- Braising requires a heavy pot. It must take the heat of the first step – the sauté and then, the simmer.

- A Dutch oven, either all metal or ceramic-clad metal, works beautifully. The pot must have a tight lid to retain the steam.

- You can finish the braising process either on top of the stove or in the oven.

- A slow cooker is not suitable unless you sauté your food first and then add it to the pot.

Stews & Meat

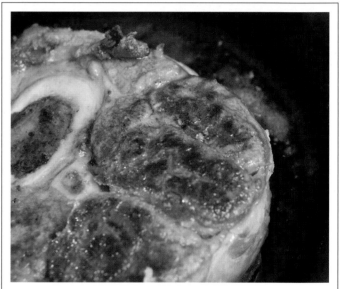

- Stews and pot roasts are braised. The beef, veal, or lamb is seared until brown. It's pushed to the side, and then the vegetables are sautéed until softened.

- The liquids are added and the heat reduced to a very slow simmer.

- The stew is covered and allowed to cook very gently until the beef is tender.

- The stew can be thickened after removing the meat and vegetables by adding quick-blending flour or a mixture of flour and water.

tough and tired. The only blast of heat you give a braised dish is at the very outset. The sear is the one short exposure to high heat. If, once you have added the liquids, you let the chili, stew, pot roast, or fricassee boil, you will create a dry, tough dinner. Add liquids as necessary, keeping an even level of wine, broth, or tomato sauce to almost cover the meat. Then, give it an occasional stir.

After browning the meat, sauté aromatic vegetables, which include garlic, onions, and parsnips, to add essential flavor to the braised dish. Adding broth and wine will create deep, rich flavors. It takes time for the wine to mellow in the gravy or sauce. Other flavors can be added as you go along or toward the end of the cooking time.

Chili

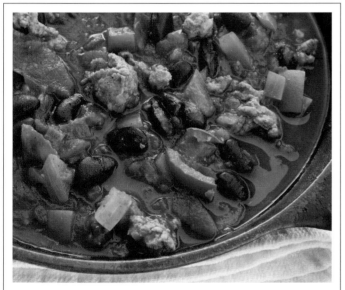

- Whether made with turkey, beef, pork, or veal, chili is braised.

- The meat is browned first. If you brown your vegetables first, they'll burn when you sauté your meat.

- The quantity and variety of vegetables can be quite a challenge, with onions, garlic, and sweet and hot peppers.

- If there's too much liquid when the chili is done, simply take the cover off and let it simmer down until it reaches the thickness you like. Timing depends on quantity of extra liquid.

Chicken

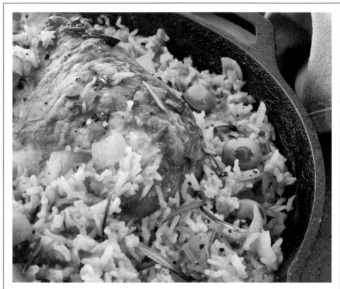

- When you braise chicken, it absorbs whatever flavors you add to the pot. The olives, herbs, garlic, and onions all are incorporated.

- The wine and olives in this recipe clearly affect the flavors of the chicken, the rice, and the liquid, which becomes sauce.

- The method of sautéing (browning) the chicken gives it a very appetizing golden color.

- The braising process makes it certain that the chicken is cooked through.

BOILING & STEAMING

These are two simple techniques that you will use often in cooking

Boiling and steaming are two basic techniques that all great cooks need to know. Boiling is used for dried foods, while steaming is usually used for vegetables and Asian rice dishes. Dried grains, legumes, and pasta are boiled because they are dried, hard, and must absorb moisture to soften enough to eat.

Boiling occurs in three stages: The first is the scald or simmer; tiny bubbles appear around the side of the pot. The

second stage is the slow boil, with gentle bubbles all over the surface of the liquid. The rolling boil is a full 212°F. All you need is a pot large enough to hold the cooking liquid.

Steaming exposes food to evaporating liquid. There are metal and bamboo steamers that you can use for this technique. The easiest steaming method is to put the food you want to steam in a glass or ceramic dish with a bit of water,

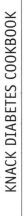

Boiling In Extra Nutrition

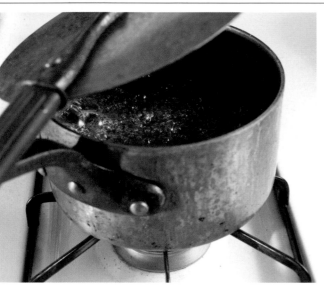

- You need a good 2- to 4-quart pot for boiling dried foods. Be sure to use a pot that's big enough for the food to fit without overflowing. It can double as a soup kettle.

- Your pot for boiling foods, such as pasta, must have two handles for gripping.

- Pasta pots with a removable colander make lifting and draining the food easier.

- When boiling polenta or rice, choose from vegetable, chicken, or beef broth to enrich flavor and nutrition.

Microwave Steaming

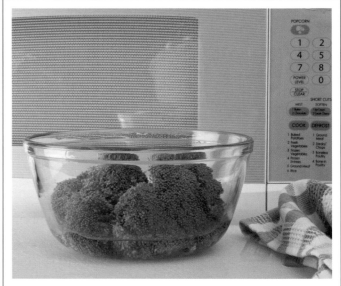

- Steamed broccoli is delicious and healthy to make. Rinse broccoli in a colander and toss in a large glass bowl with lemon juice.

- A Pyrex bowl is excellent for microwave steaming. You can put a lot of broccoli in the bowl.

- The veggies are steamed in the microwave. Then they are finished in the sauce.

- Stock up on freezer paper or waxed paper – either works fine for wrapping a bowl of vegetables to be microwaved.

cover it with paper, and place it in the microwave. Depending on the quantity of vegetables and whether you like them crisp-tender or soft, time will vary from 1 minute to 3 or 4 minutes.

So how do you know when to boil and when to steam? Boil vegetables only in soup. The reason for not boiling vegetables to be served at the table is that a great many of the nutrients end up in the water, not in the food. If vegetables are cooked in the soup, the goodness goes into the cooking liquid, not down the drain.

Carrots, broccoli, cauliflower, and other stiff vegetables, are best steamed in the microwave. Rinsed spinach that's moist actually steams as it is sautéed in olive oil. Bitter greens such as kale and broccoli rabe are blanched, dropped in boiling water for a few seconds, then drained and sautéed. Frozen vegetables are best when microwaved. Many are sold in pouches with timing instructions. Whole artichokes are the exception; they are best boiled.

Presteaming Vegetables

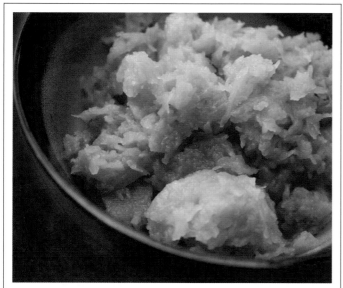

- The presteaming technique covers butternut squash, turban squash, and pumpkins.

- Winter squash is presteamed in the microwave prior to stuffing and roasting or mashing.

- You don't have to cut it in half; simply make slits with a knife so the steam can come out.

- Once the squash is steamed in the microwave, it can be cut up and mashed, cut in half and stuffed, or baked.

Steaming on the Stove

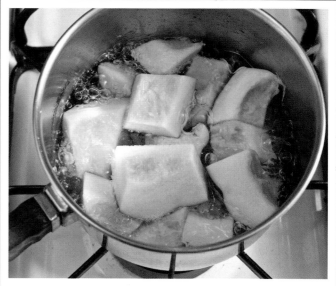

- When beans are steamed in a pot, the lid must be tight, or the beans will dry out and burn.

- You need a good, heavy-bottomed saucepan or pot for steaming.

- Metal steamers that adapt to the size of the pot are useful, as they keep the vegetables off the bottom of the pan.

- Adjust the timing of the steaming to the size and fatness of the beans. You can always pull one out and test it.

BAKING DISHES & PANS

A few square and round glass and ceramic pans are multifunctional in your kitchen

Certain metal and most glass dishes and pans are excellent for baking, whether it's a delectable dessert or a hearty entrée. Casseroles are baked in 1- to 2-quart ceramic or glass containers, most with lids, whereas many pasta and cheese dishes are baked in rectangular glass pans measuring 9 inches by 13 inches. And, of course, a cookie sheet is an essential part

of any kitchen for far more than cookies.

Pyrex and CorningWare baking dishes go from the freezer to the microwave for defrosting or to the oven for baking. They are excellent for casseroles that you can make in advance and then bake for dinner. Use heavy-bottomed pots on top of the stove to start your aromatic vegetables, boil potatoes, etc.

Casserole Dishes

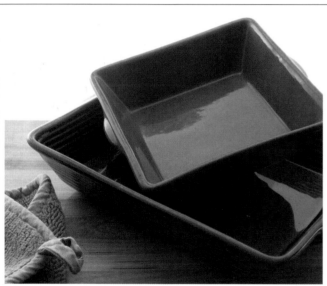

- Depending on their size, bake egg dishes in a large ceramic gratin dish or a rectangular lasagna pan. Recipes with eggs in them will puff up nicely.

- Casserole dishes can go in the microwave as well as the dishwasher.

- Be careful, however; some Pyrex will break if heated to 450°F.

- Egg casseroles, when made in casserole dishes, can be prepared a day in advance, refrigerated, and baked just before serving.

Glass Baking Dishes

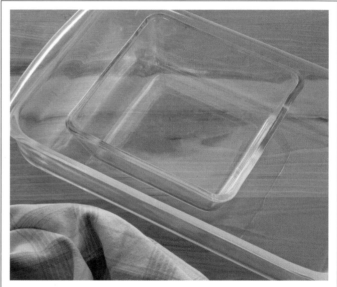

- When baking, use glass baking dishes that will withstand a high temperature in the oven.

- Baked fruit, for example, is best made in these types of dishes. Try baking individual portions of fruit in glass custard cups.

- Most baking takes place at 325 to 350°F. Any hotter is likely to burn the food.

- Baking at below 325°F will dry out the food and take forever to cook.

A flat-bottomed, straight-sided soufflé dish is essential to the pumpkin soufflé recipe in the dessert section but can also be used for other wonderful dessert dishes. You'll find that your baking dishes are multipurpose. When you acquire kitchen equipment, buy multipurpose pots, pans, muffin tins, and dishes. These can be found directly from manufacturer Web sites or at various discount stores. Many upscale department stores and culinary stores also have kitchen departments that offer cooking classes.

Cookie Sheets

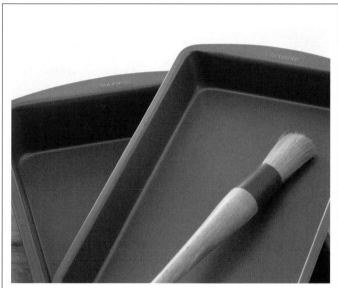

- Cookie sheets are great multipurpose dishes to use in the kitchen, and there is a wide variety of foods that can be cooked on them.

- Meringue tarts, for example, do well when on cookie sheets. They typically bake for a long time on low heat.

- Meringues can be baked on a flat cookie sheet to make small, individual tarts.

- Individual meringue tarts are piped onto the cookie sheet through a pastry bag or heavy plastic bag.

Soufflé Dishes

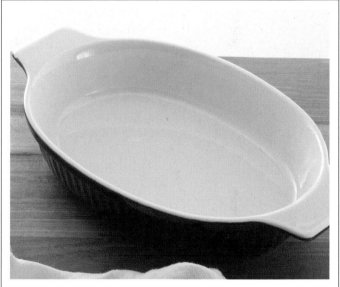

- To ensure a puffed soufflé, as opposed to a "sou-flop," you need a real soufflé dish. These dishes come in various sizes and individual portion sizes, too.

- For a soufflé, preheat the oven to 400°F so that the egg whites get a blast of heat at the outset.

- After 15 minutes, turn the oven temperature down to 325°F.

- The soufflé dish uniformly distributes heat, and its high sides ensure that none of the gooey deliciousness of the dish falls out.

TECHNIQUES

BROILING & GRILLING

Use these essential techniques when cooking fish and meat

Broiling and grilling are two techniques you will use often in the kitchen, and sometimes outdoors, on either a charcoal or gas grill. These two techniques operate differently to produce tasty and flavorful results. Broiling supplies flame from above, while grilling supplies it from below. Broiling employs gas or electricity; grilling uses gas, wood, or charcoal. Broiling can be a great cooking technique to use when you are trying to stick to a calorie-controlled diet, as much of the calorie-rich meat fat drips away during the cooking process.

Many kitchens are equipped with open-flame grills. Some may have charcoal-burning elements with excellent hoods to suck out the fumes. Never bring a charcoal grill indoors unless you have the proper venting equipment. Propane gas grills should not be brought indoors, even if it's raining

Broiling

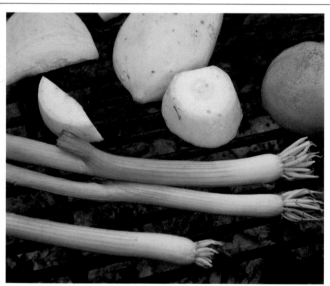

- Broiling sends the heat from the top down to the food. Set your oven on broil. If you want to sear the food, set the temperature 400°F to 500°F.

- To broil the food slowly, as with a thick piece of meat

or fish, set the temperature between 300°F to 400°F.

- Another method of slow broiling is to move the rack down to a lower slot, between four and twelve inches from the flame.

Grilling

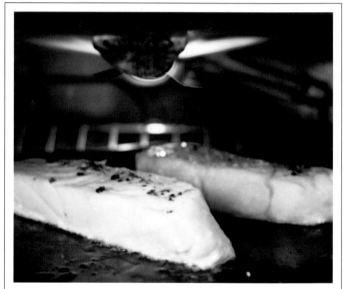

- Grill your fish in- or out-doors. The stove-top grill is useful for burgers and steaks. With grilling, heat comes from the bottom up.

- Stovetop grills are generally wrought iron or enamel-coated metal. You can control heat for searing and for slower cooking.

- When using a charcoal grill, you need to get used to letting it develop until the coals are a soft rose in color with a light coating of ash, not flaring.

- Simply set a gas grill to the desired temperature, high for searing, and medium to cook food through.

outside. Carbon monoxide is a very dangerous, potentially deadly gas, and any kind of flame produces this gas, so keep your stove hood fan working whenever you grill or broil.

Oven broiling employs the use of enamel or nonstick-coated metal pans. These pans should have racks to keep the meat off the bottom of the pan. Preheat your broiler before cooking in order to get the food cooked through. With a thick piece of meat or fish, sear it first on both sides to brown. Then, turn the oven to bake mode to finish internal cooking.

Broiling Food

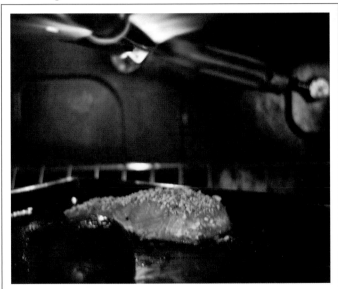

- Keep your broiler, grill, and oven very clean. Clean them often. You do not want a buildup of grease to taint the flavors of your food or start a fire in your oven.

- Cover broiler pans with aluminum foil. Use nonstick spray on top of the foil.

- As soon as your outdoor grill is cool and you've finished dinner, spray it with a degreaser and rub it down with a wire brush.

- Be sure to keep food at least six inches from the flame.

Timing

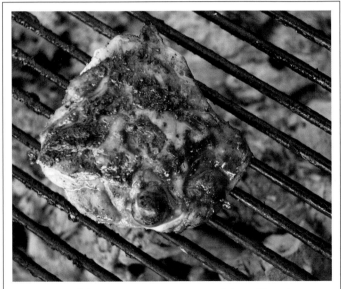

- Timing is of the essence when broiling or grilling. A meat thermometer is far more reliable than a timer.

- Timing varies according to how you like your food done.

- If the food browns too fast, change oven to the baking mode, lower the temperature of the grill, and cover the meat.

- Bone-in and skin-on meats will take longer to cook than boneless and skinless meat.

- Chicken can dry out quickly on the grill or in the broiler. Always watch food you broil or grill carefully.

TECHNIQUES

ROASTING
Learn these techniques to help you cook a variety of healthy foods

Terms can get confusing when it comes to roasting. A roast is generally a large piece of meat or a whole chicken, turkey, duck, or pheasant. But a pot roast is braised meat, browned and then slowly simmered in a liquid until it is very well done. A round roast, rib roast, or top sirloin of beef may be basted but cooks in the oven uncovered; beef or lamb is often served rare to medium.

The best technique for roasting a meat is to start cooking it on high, and then reduce the heat to let it cook through. This is true of oven roasts of beef, lamb, and pork roasts. A pork roast with the bone in should also get a flash of heat to sear it, and then the heat should be lowered until the meat is done. The reverse is true of a large turkey. It should be covered and cooked slowly until the end, and then be uncovered to brown.

Lamb Roasts

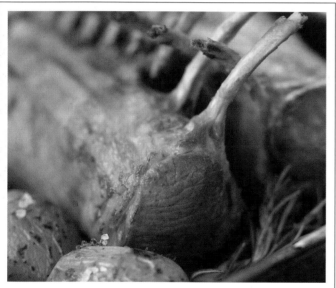

- With a lamb roast, you need to cut virtually all of the fat off of the meat. The fat is strong and will ruin the flavor of the meat.

- If you can get young lamb, it's much better in flavor than a mature sheep, known as mutton.

- Marinating the lamb tenderizes it.

- Baby rack of lamb doesn't need marinating and needs very little trimming. It's broiled and then baked.

Roasting Equipment

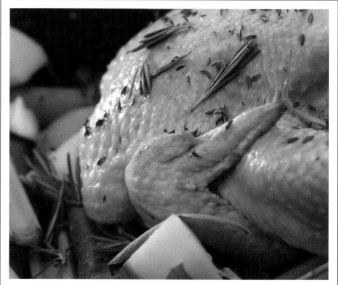

- The equipment you need is simple. If you can't spend for a really great roaster, use an aluminum foil one.

- Meat thermometers also come in handy when cooking meat. Some thermometers are built into the oven, and others sit on the top of the oven, connected to the meat with a long cord.

- Use aluminum foil or heavy kitchen towels to rest the meat. This step is essential. If the meat does not rest, the juices will run out when it's carved. When it's rested, the juice returns to the meat.

Essential equipment for roasting includes an enamel-covered metal roasting pan with a rack, or a disposable aluminum one, and a meat thermometer.

Roasting Large Food

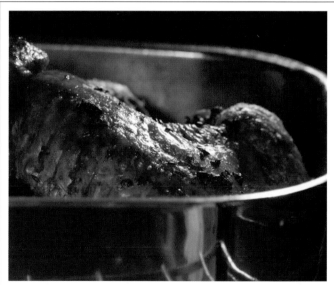

- In the case of a large rib roast or turkey, you may need to "tent" it with aluminum foil to ensure that it will be cooked through.

- Tenting prevents meat from drying out and browning. Remove tents when meat is 30 minutes from being done so that it browns.

- Some cooks start turkeys, chickens, ducks, and geese breast-down on a bed of celery and carrots. This sends juices into the breast.

- When roasting small birds such as ducks, game hens, or quail, wrap the drumsticks in foil to keep them from drying out.

Basting

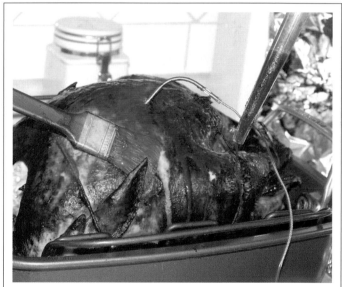

- Basting, or adding liquid to the meat, is an important technique in roasting. Use a variety of liquids or a mixture. For example, use chicken or vegetable broth on chicken.

- A mixture of red wine and beef broth works well on filet mignon and rib, round, or top sirloin roasts.

- Herbs make a tasty addition to basting liquid. Add 1 tablespoon of rosemary to your chicken baste; add 1 teaspoon of sage leaves to your beef.

- Use a bulb basting tool, a small ladle, or a pastry brush.

TECHNIQUES

FAMILY FRITTATA

A frittata can be served hot, cold, or at room temperature

A frittata is an Italian open-faced omelet. It is versatile and delicious. Making a frittata is easier than making an omelet because you don't have to worry about it sticking or having to fold it in half.

This frittata is stuffed with caramelized onions, fresh tomatoes, and basil. You can stuff a frittata with mushrooms or a combination of cheeses, and thinly sliced Italian sausages and favorite herbs can be added. Try a frittata with fresh baby spinach or frozen spinach and Gorgonzola cheese.

Kids love frittata, as do adults; they are a great way to use up the leftovers in your refrigerator. Chop some cooked leftover broccoli, add cheese and eggs, and you've got lunch. *Yield: 8 servings*

Ingredients

2 tablespoons olive oil

1 whole sweet onion, white or yellow, peeled and thinly sliced

5 whole eggs

4 egg whites

Freshly ground black pepper to taste

1/3 cup grated Parmesan cheese

1/4 teaspoon salt (optional)

1 medium tomato, core removed, and thinly sliced

10 large basil leaves, shredded, or 1 teaspoon dried basil

Calories 109, **Fat** (g) 8, **Carbohydrates** (g) 2, **Protein** (g) 8, **Fiber** (g) 0, **Saturated Fat** (g) 2, **Cholesterol** (mg) 136, **Sodium** (mg) 136, **ADA Exchange** 1 lean meat, 1 fat

Family Frittata

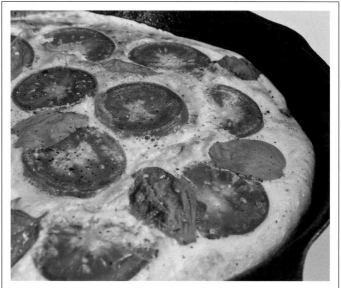

- Heat oil over low heat in a large cast-iron pan. Add onions. Cook until softened. Remove from heat.

- Place eggs and whites in a blender with pepper and Parmesan cheese. Add salt, if desired. Blend until smooth. Pour over onions and stir to distribute evenly.

- Arrange tomatoes and basil over the top. Place on low heat and cook until well set. Leave it a bit runny on top.

- Place under the broiler until lightly browned, about two minutes. Cut into wedges and serve.

By cutting the number of egg yolks and using more egg whites, you reduce the calories and cholesterol drastically. Using nonstick spray rather than oil also cuts down on your fat intake. You can also use egg substitutes and other low-fat ingredients, such as mushrooms, spinach, herbs, tomatoes, and other vegetables. Try adding grilled vegetables for a wonderful boost.

• • • • RECIPE VARIATION • • • •

Try new flavors: Experiment with dill and salmon as ingredients in your frittata for a flavorful punch. Or add some rosemary and ½ cup crumbled turkey bacon. Fruit can be added to a frittata if you are making it for dessert. Use the basic egg recipe and add ½ cup sliced peaches and berries. Sprinkle the top with Splenda when the frittata is done.

Cast-Iron Frying Pans

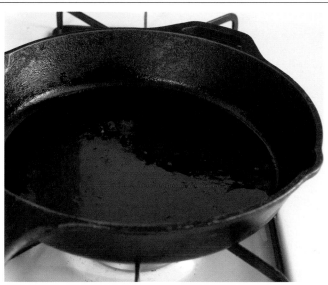

Seasoning Cast-Iron Pans

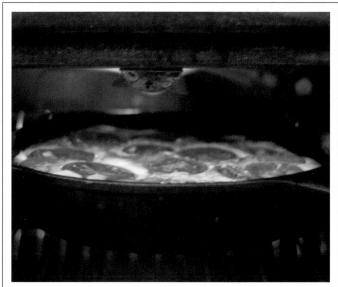

- Cast-iron pans are good for more than frying. Black and heavy, they are wonderful for all kinds of cooking. They hold the heat and distribute it evenly.

- These pans are perfect for using in the broiler to brown food before serving. You can't do this with

any pan that has a plastic handle.

- Be careful, however; use a potholder when picking up a hot cast-iron pan.

- Use cast-iron pans to make pancakes, simmer stew, or fry chicken.

- These pans must be seasoned before using. First, heat the pan; then remove it from the heat and add cooking oil (not olive oil!)

- Let the oil soak in while the pan cools, and then wipe it off with paper towels.

- Once the pan is seasoned, don't wash it with detergent or you will have to reseason it.

- Just rinse the pan in hot water and wipe it dry with a paper towel after each use. You will have to reseason it occasionally.

PUFFY EGG WHITE OMELET

One bite and you'll be a believer in the "incredible, edible egg"

Egg white omelets are delicious, simple, and incredibly versatile. They cut absolutely all of the cholesterol out of the eggs.

This recipe is for a puffed omelet. However, you can also make it traditionally. Avoid the "puff" by maintaining a gentle whisk of the eggs.

This omelet, filled with lemon-flavored ricotta and spinach, has a delightful tangy flavor. To prep, thaw the spinach completely, making sure to squeeze all of the extra moisture out of the spinach. Or, make your filling with a couple of handfuls of fresh baby spinach, chopped and mixed in with the ricotta. *Yield: 4 servings*

Ingredients

1 cup low-fat ricotta cheese

1 (10-ounce) box frozen chopped spinach or 1 cup fresh baby spinach, chopped and packed

$^1/_4$ teaspoon ground nutmeg

1 teaspoon lemon zest

$^1/_4$ cup Parmesan cheese

10 egg whites

Calories 173, **Fat** (g) 7, **Carbohydrates** (g) 7, **Protein** (g) 21, **Fiber** (g) 2, **Saturated Fat** (g) 4, **Cholesterol** (mg) 25, **Sodium** (mg) 263, **ADA Exchange** 1 vegetable, 3 lean meat

Puffy Egg White Omelet

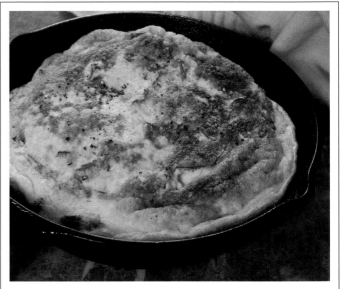

- Mix ricotta, spinach, nutmeg, lemon zest, and Parmesan cheese in a bowl.

- Beat or whisk egg whites until they form high peaks; add salt, if desired. Fold ricotta-spinach mixture into egg whites.

- Preheat broiler. Spray a large cast-iron frying pan with nonstick spray.

- Place pan over medium heat. Add egg mixture. Don't stir. Cook until mixture starts to brown on the sides. Place under the broiler to brown the top, about two minutes.

Puff and fill that omelet: You can get a nice puff going for your omelet by beating the egg whites with an eggbeater or whisk. Fill the omelet by folding the goodies into the egg white mixture. For the full puff, start your omelet in a nonstick pan on top of the stove and then finish it in the oven.

• • • • RECIPE VARIATION • • • •

Add a bit of greenery: In addition to spinach, you can add chopped cooked broccoli, arugula, or a combination of tomatoes and herbs. Another great filling for any omelet is asparagus, cooked and cut into one-inch pieces. Or if you're splurging, just use the tips (save the rest of the spears for soup).

Separating Egg Whites

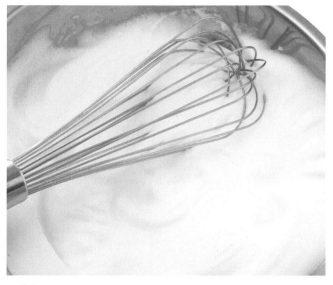

Working with the Broiler

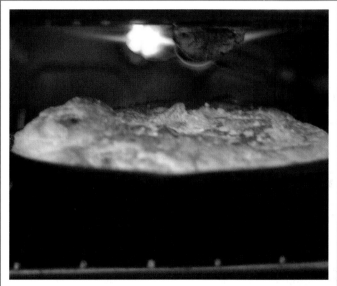

- If there is even a speck of egg yolk mixed with the whites, they will not whip properly.

- They will be foamy but not "peaky," puffy, or perky. Be sure your whisk or eggbeater blades are completely degreased and clean.

- When you separate more than one or two eggs, it's smart to use two glass bowls, one for the yolks and the other for the whites.

- Separate egg whites individually into a large bowl so that you can check for yolk.

- Often a recipe requires more than just a pass on top of the stove, which only cooks the bottom of the food.

- You will have to run the pan under the broiler.

- Be vigilant with the broiler. It's easy to burn the top of a dish and leave the inside raw.

- If the top is golden and it's only been in for a moment, turn off the broiler, close the oven door, and let it cook with low heat for a few more minutes.

HALF-YOLK OMELET WITH SALSA

This is a wonderful way to retain the rich "eggy" flavor while cutting the fat

You can make this recipe either in two batches, each serving two, or as one big omelet to serve four. Using two nonstick pans makes it easy to do two at the same time.

Just be sure to prepare and place your fillings on the side of the stove before you start to cook the eggs. As soon as the omelets begin to set, you can add the fillings and fold the omelets in half to finish cooking.

Some people like their omelets soft and runny, while others like them well-set, almost stiff. It's simply a matter of timing. Just be sure to reduce the heat so that you don't burn the bottom of the more "done" omelet. *Yield: 4 servings*

KNACK DIABETES COOKBOOK

Ingredients

4 whole eggs

6 egg whites

³/₄ cup fresh tomato salsa (mild, medium, or hot, to taste)

¹/₂ cup low-fat cheddar cheese, shredded

4 tablespoons low-fat sour cream

Calories 157, **Fat** (g) 8, **Carbohydrates** (g) 5, **Protein** (g) 16, **Fiber** (g) 1, **Saturated Fat** (g) 3, **Cholesterol** (mg) 220, **Sodium** (mg) 536, **ADA Exchange** 2 lean meat

Half-Yolk Omelet with Salsa

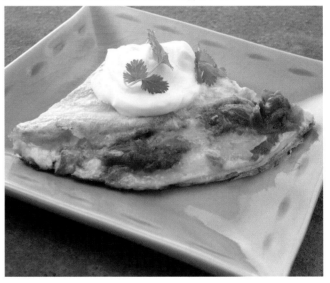

- Break whole eggs into a bowl. Add whites to the whole eggs. Whisk eggs until well blended.

- Prepare a 10-inch nonstick pan with nonstick spray. Or, prepare two (7-inch) pans the same way.

- Pour eggs in the pan(s);

tip to spread eggs evenly. When top sets, spoon salsa on one side and sprinkle with cheese.

- Fold half of the omelet(s) over salsa and cheese. Slip onto a plate and divide into servings. Spoon sour cream over top of each serving.

Brunch, lunch, or supper omelets: An omelet can be as full of food or as light as you wish—perfect for any meal. A medium-light omelet contains two whites for each yolk (e.g., four egg whites to two yolks), as opposed to all whole eggs. A light omelet consists of all egg whites. For light omelets for big meals, try fruit fillings, low-fat cheese, and/or light meats, such as 2 ounces per person of smoked turkey or turkey sausage. Add ¼ cup baby shrimp for a flavorful lunch omelet. You can add asparagus, chopped artichoke hearts, and roasted vegetables. If you serve an omelet for brunch or lunch, add a side salad to keep it light. If it's a supper omelet, start with soup and serve hot multigrain bread on the side.

Don't Let It Dry Out

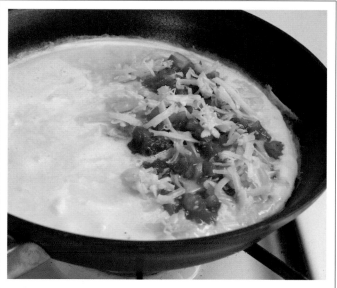

- If your omelet gets too dry, it will crack and be difficult to fold. To avoid this, place the filling on one side, then immediately turn the plain side onto the filled side.

- Or, spoon the filling down the middle of the omelet, and then fold each side over the middle.

- Next, turn the omelet over, leaving the smooth side on top. This melds the sides together.

- Carefully remove the omelet to a warm platter. Cut into serving pieces and add extra salsa to each.

A Kitchen Sink Omelet

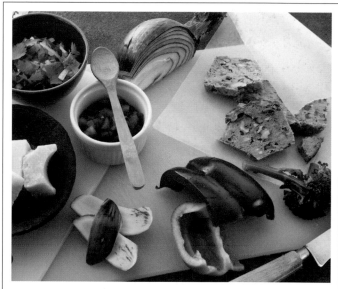

- When you're home alone, an omelet becomes the ultimate comfort food. It's a snap to make, and it's also easy on the digestive system.

- Try making a "kitchen sink" omelet from leftovers. Start with an inventory of your fridge and freezer.

- Leftover veggies from a salad work well, as do leftover cold cuts, steak, chicken, or uncooked shrimp.

- Use bits of cheese and whatever else is in there. Whisk up a couple of eggs or one whole egg and two whites.

EGGS & DAIRY

SALMON & EGG CASSEROLE

With this do-ahead dish, you can plan on a leisurely brunch

The delicious combination of salmon, cream cheese, eggs, and scallions makes a fabulous dish for friends and family.

Put this recipe together the day or night before for a quick meal. Pop it in the oven just before your company arrives, and relax. It is best baked in a large oval gratin pan or dish, either copper-clad or ceramic, which gives you a lot of surface to brown. You can use multigrain white bread or a

multigrain baguette instead of sourdough.

Another important point about this recipe is that it tastes far richer and more caloric than it really is. Serve it with a crisp green salad on the side, or toss half a box of frozen petit pois (very small green peas) into the casserole before baking. *Yield: 8 servings*

Ingredients

2 cups low-fat or fat-free milk

10 eggs

1 teaspoon homemade mustard (see recipe, page 208) or dry English mustard

¹/₂ teaspoon cayenne pepper

8 ounces low-fat or light cream cheese, in chunks

1 loaf multigrain sourdough French bread, (two inches in diameter) cut in ³/₄-inch cubes

1 bunch scallions with roots removed, chopped into ¹/₄-inch pieces

¹/₄ pound smoked salmon (Irish if available), available at any supermarket

Freshly ground black pepper to taste

Calories 325, **Fat** (g) 8, **Carbohydrates** (g) 43, **Protein** (g) 20, **Fiber** (g) 5, **Saturated Fat** (g) 4, **Cholesterol** (mg) 21, **Sodium** (mg) 709, **Carb Choices** 2½, **ADA Exchange** 2 starch, ½ milk, 1½ meat, 1 fat

Salmon & Egg Casserole

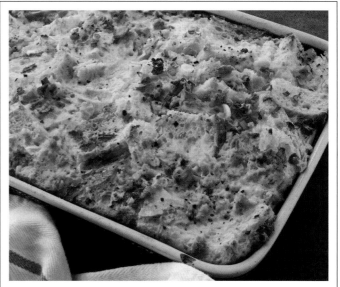

- Process milk, eggs, mustard, and cayenne in blender for 1 minute. With blender on low, add cream cheese 1 teaspoonful at a time.

- Prepare casserole dish with nonstick spray. Spread in bread cubes. Pour in milk, egg, and cheese mixture. Cover; refrigerate overnight.

- Remove from fridge 30 minutes before baking. Preheat oven to 350°F. Mix scallions and salmon into bread mixture.

- Sprinkle with black pepper; bake 1 hour or until puffed and golden. Serve immediately.

Added nutrients: The multigrain sourdough bread provides fiber, B vitamins, and other nutrients that are good for the diet. Serve the casserole with a side salad of roasted beets and greens. Or, make a traditional Greek salad, but with only half of the feta cheese, as there is plenty of cheese in the casserole.

• • • • RECIPE VARIATION • • • •

For a different taste: Replace salmon with the same quantity of ham, smoked turkey, cooked turkey bacon, or cooked Italian or American turkey sausage. Use 2 cups of shredded, low-fat cheddar or ricotta rather than cream cheese. Thaw and drain a package of frozen spinach to add, or use 2 cups fresh spinach and roasted red pepper or green pepper for added nutrients.

Blender Secrets

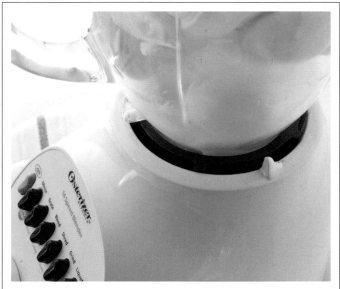

- Always start blending with the recipe's liquids and make sure they are completely mixed; this can take about two minutes.

- When adding flour, cheese, or sugar, do so slowly, with the motor on low.

- In between additions, give the liquids time to "digest" the more solid ingredients.

- Be sure to turn the machine off from time to time and scrape the sides with a rubber spatula. This ensures that everything is completely blended.

Proper Dishes for Fridge and Oven

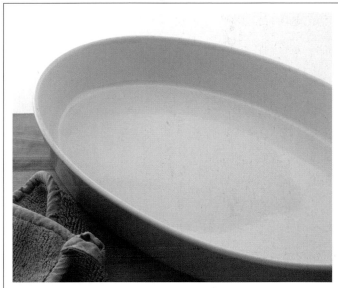

- Some manufacturers claim that their containers can go from the refrigerator or freezer straight into a preheated oven.

- This isn't a good idea. The food will cook more evenly if it isn't frozen or icy cold.

- Ceramic or glass casserole dishes can crack or even break in half, neither of which you want to have happen to your delicious casserole.

- Be sure you use dishes that can sustain both heat and cold.

CLAFOUTI WITH PEACHES & HAM

This classic French dessert can be adapted for a special breakfast or brunch

Traditionally, clafoutis are made with fresh, pitted cherries and a lot more sugar than in this recipe. You'll find that you can use Splenda, or eliminate most of the sugar entirely. Instead of cherries, we suggest peaches. The peaches should be blanched, peeled, pitted, and sliced. You can use just about any fruit you like, however, and the ham is optional.

The dish looks very pretty baked in a white or decorated ceramic pie pan.

With this particular recipe, you get your dairy, carbs, and protein in one dish. You can also sauce it with some fresh fruit compote, a dollop of low-fat sour cream, or a small scoop of sorbet for added flavor. *Yield: 6 servings*

Ingredients

1 cup low-fat milk

2 tablespoons Splenda for baking

5 eggs or egg substitute

1 teaspoon vanilla extract

1/2 teaspoon salt

2/3 cup all-purpose flour

4 large or 6 small peaches, blanched, peeled, and cut into slices

1/4 pound low-sodium smoked or boiled ham, thinly sliced and shredded

Calories 204, **Fat** (g) 7, **Carbohydrates** (g) 23, **Protein** (g) 13, **Fiber** (g) 2, **Saturated Fat** (g) 2, **Cholesterol** (mg) 189, **Sodium** (mg) 454, **Carb Choices** 1½, **ADA Exchange** 1½ fruit, 2 lean meat

Clafouti with Peaches & Ham

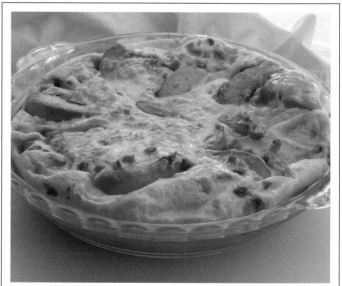

- Preheat oven to 350°F. Mix milk, Splenda, eggs, vanilla, salt, and flour in blender until smooth, about 2 minutes.

- Prepare a glass or ceramic pie pan with nonstick spray. Pour ¼ inch of batter into the pan; place it over very low flame.

- When it has set, add the peaches and ham, distributing them evenly on top.

- Pour the rest of the batter in the pan; bake in oven on middle rack about 30 minutes, until golden brown and puffed. Cut into wedges.

MAKE IT EASY

Local farm stands or green markets are a great source of fresh food that can be enjoyed year-round. It doesn't take long to blanch, peel, and freeze a peck of peaches for winter pies; just add a bit of lemon juice and 1 teaspoon of sugar to the freezer container. You can then have fresh peach pies, clafoutis, or omelets during the chilly months.

Blanching Fruit for Easy Peeling

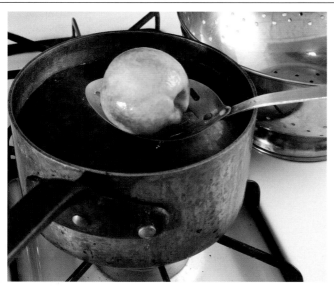

Slicing Blanched Fruit

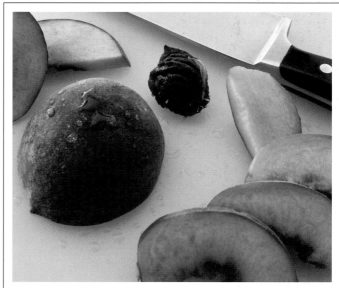

- Bring a large pot of water to a boil.

- Lower the fruit (peaches, apricots, nectarines) gently into the water. Turn the fruit to immerse fully.

- In about 2 minutes, remove the fruit. Place it in a colan-der and let cool so you can handle it. Cold water can be run over the fruit to speed cooling and stop the cooking process.

- Slip off the skins. Cut the fruit in half; remove pits and slice.

- Rather than holding a slippery piece of blanched fruit in your hand, try this:

- Cut fruit in half. Remove the pit.

- Place cut-side down on a chopping board. Using a very sharp paring knife, slice lengthwise and place in a bowl.

- Add 1 teaspoon of lemon juice to the fruit to prevent it from turning brown. Use the same technique for preparing fresh fruit to be frozen.

WORLD-CLASS SCRAMBLED EGGS

Your friends and family will want to know the secret to this dish

My mother brought this recipe home from a visit to the Scottish Highlands in the 1960s. She loved the scrambled eggs prepared this way, and couldn't believe how easy, simple, and special the recipe was.

Ever since she gave me the recipe, I've been dong scrambled eggs in this way. People always ask for my secret.

It's simply a different formula: same fresh eggs, but much more milk than you'd ordinarily use, and a very different and far gentler handling when the eggs are in the pan. The results are truly amazing. *Yield: 4 servings*

Ingredients

6 whole eggs

3 egg whites

²/₃ cup low-fat milk

Salt to taste

Freshly ground black pepper to taste

1 tablespoon butter or olive oil

Calories 166, **Fat** (g) 11, **Carbohydrates** (g) 3, **Protein** (g) 14, **Fiber** (g) 0, **Saturated Fat** (g) 4, **Cholesterol** (mg) 327, **Sodium** (mg) 164, **ADA Exchange** 2 lean meat, 1 fat

World-Class Scrambled Eggs

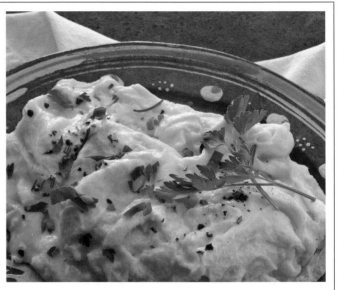

- Whisk or use an eggbeater to blend the whole eggs, egg whites, milk, salt, and pepper. Prepare a nonstick pan with nonstick spray, oil, or butter (melted in pan).

- Place pan over medium-high heat. Add the eggs and reduce the heat to low.

- Let the eggs start to set, and then gently fold the eggs, once only, going around the sides of the pan with a rubber spatula.

- Cook to desired doneness and serve.

Embellishing your eggs: Eggs au naturel is a popular way to serve this dish; however, you can enhance it with lots of different goodies. When eggs are almost done, add ½ cup chopped herbs. Or, add one-half cup of crumbled Gorgonzola or Parmesan cheese. You can also add ½ cup chopped tomatoes, caramelized onions, bits of smoked turkey, or low-salt ham. One-half cup of roasted red peppers, minced, brightens up the eggs. A half cup of chopped, chunky fresh mozzarella makes them chewy, while strips of white American cheese melt beautifully and give the eggs a creamy touch. One (14-ounce) can of unmarinated artichokes adds a lot of interest. Add blanched and drained asparagus tips combined with 1 teaspoon of lemon zest.

Adding Herbs

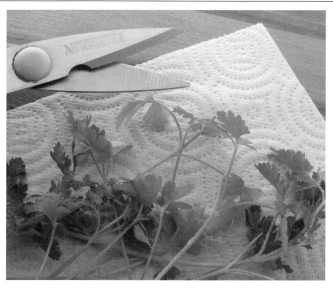

Keeping Hot Food Hot

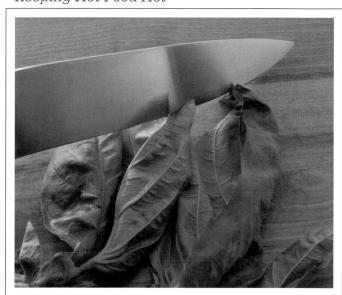

- Fresh herbs and eggs go very well together. Rather than mixing herbs into the eggs before cooking, try this method:

- Rinse and dry a bunch of fresh Italian flat-leaf parsley, a bunch of chives, and two or three sprigs of fresh oregano and basil leaves.

- Remove leaves from stems. Using kitchen shears, snip the parsley and chives onto a piece of waxed paper; add the oregano leaves and tear the basil. Sprinkle over eggs.

- Cold scrambled eggs are not appealing. In the wintertime, warm the plates either on a hot tray or in a slow oven for a few minutes so that the eggs won't pick up a chill from the plates.

- If you are making a large batch for a crowd, be sure to undercook the eggs slightly and keep them on a warm platter.

- The longer eggs sit out, the more done they will get if kept on a hot tray.

EGGS & DAIRY

47

BASIC CREPES
Fabulous and easy to make, these crepes can be savory or sweet

Crepes are wonderful for most any meal, whether it's a light lunch or a quick snack. They're great either sweet or savory, whatever you desire.

Sweet crepes can be filled with anything you like, including almost any fruit and/or creamy pudding. They are festive when filled with slightly cooked berries.

Savory crepes filled with asparagus and dressed with a warm mayonnaise and cheese sauce are delicious for brunch. They can be stuffed with spinach and ricotta cheese or chicken and mushrooms.

You can make crepes a maximum of three days ahead of time and keep them in the refrigerator, or you can make them one week ahead and freeze them. *Yield: 4 servings (3 6-inch crepes per serving)*

Ingredients:

For the crepes:

2 cups cold fat-free milk

2 whole eggs

3 egg whites

1/2 teaspoon salt

2 tablespoons Splenda (only if making sweet crepes)

1 1/2 cups all-purpose flour

1/2 cup whole-wheat flour

2 tablespoons unsalted butter

1 tablespoon low-fat margarine

For the filling (sweet crepes):

1/2 cup cold water

1 tablespoon cornstarch

1 teaspoon Splenda

1 cup fresh raspberries

1 1/2 cups fresh blueberries

Calories 422, **Fat** (g) 10, **Carbohydrates** (g) 67, **Protein** (g) 18, **Fiber** (g) 6, **Saturated Fat** (g) 5, **Cholesterol** (mg) 124, **Sodium** (mg) 443, **Carb Choices** 4½, **ADA Exchange** ½ fat-free milk, 2 starch, 2 fruit, 1 medium-fat meat, 1 fat

Basic Crepes

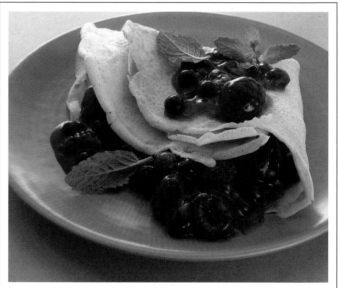

- Blend milk, eggs, salt, and Splenda. On low, slowly add flour. Scrape bowl. Add butter, margarine; blend 1 minute. Refrigerate 2 hours.

- Heat a nonstick 7- to 9-inch pan over medium-high heat. Prepare with nonstick spray. Skim pan with ¼ cup batter to make 6-inch crepe.

- When brown, place crepes on waxed paper.

- Whisk cold water, cornstarch, and Splenda in a saucepan, and add the berries. Boil, stirring until thickened.

- Spoon berries on crepes; fold, roll. Pour juice over all.

Stuffing for savory crepes: By omitting the Splenda, you have a perfect crepe for chicken or other stuffing. Mix together 1 10-ounce can low-fat cream of chicken soup with ½ pound low-salt chicken from the deli, cut thickly and diced. Add ¼ cup Parmesan cheese and enough fat-free milk to make a thick filling. Place 2 tablespoons of the filling in the middle of a crepe. Fold and roll carefully into a tube and place in a baking pan, seam side down. Thin the rest of the sauce with more milk and pour over the top. Bake at 325°F until steaming hot and serve. Or mix ½ cup each of ricotta and spinach, and 1 egg with 1 tablespoon of Parmesan, and stuff savory crepes. You can sauce these crepes with low-fat cream of chicken soup.

How to Skim the Batter

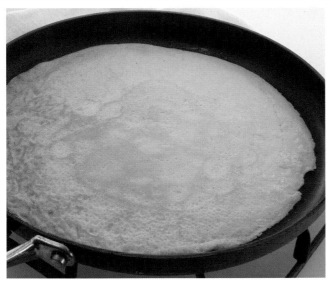

- Before heating the pan, prepare it with nonstick spray.

- Use a ladle, half full, to pour batter into the hot pan. When you add batter to the pan, lift the pan off the heat and keep moving the batter around the bottom to distribute it evenly.

- Lift the edges of the crepe with a heat-resistant spatula to prevent it from sticking. Turn the crepe as soon as it is lightly browned on the bottom. It may develop brown spots on the first side that is cooked.

Storing Crepes

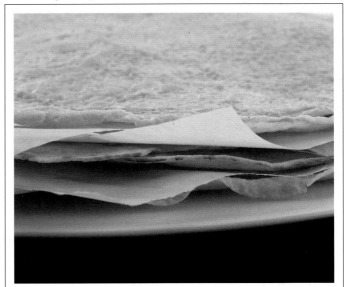

- After you cook the crepes, remove them from the pan and place each crepe on an individual sheet of waxed paper and let cool.

- Place the crepes in a sealed bag and refrigerate. If you are freezing them, make a double recipe and freeze in groups of six.

- Remember, they will be brittle when frozen, so be sure to place paper plates between the packages of crepes to be frozen to prevent them from breaking.

SPINACH-APPLE YOGURT SMOOTHIES

At breakfast or snack time, this quick smoothie can easily be part of a healthy eating plan

Smoothies can start your day with a real boost, giving you enough nourishment to last until lunch, even a late lunch. Since they can be high in carbs, try to work them into your diet plan ahead of time.

With smoothies, you can pack a bunch of healthy ingredients into one flavorful punch. Sneak cooked carrots or 1 cup of cauliflower into an orange-banana smoothie, and add a generous scoop of lemon-flavored yogurt. Look for Greek yogurt, which is lower in carbs. Or, add a handful of fresh baby spinach to a blueberry-lemon smoothie for a delightful hidden veggie mixture. *Yield: 2 servings*

KNACK DIABETES COOKBOOK

Ingredients

1 1/2 cups plain nonfat yogurt

2 tart apples

1 cup fresh spinach leaves, rinsed

1-inch piece fresh gingerroot, peeled and minced

2 tablespoons unprocessed bran

Juice of 1/2 lemon

Salt to taste

2 ice cubes, crushed

Spinach-Apple Yogurt Smoothies

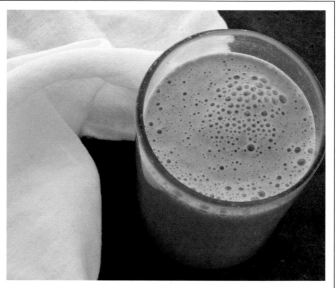

- Place all ingredients in a blender.

- Whirl until very smooth, stopping occasionally to scrape down the sides of the blender.

- Add three to four ice cubes for extra crushed ice. Add one cube at a time, to desired coldness.

Calories 203, **Fat** (g) 3, **Carbohydrates** (g) 36, **Protein** (g) 12, **Fiber** (g) 5, **Saturated Fat** (g) 2, **Cholesterol** (mg) 11, **Sodium** (mg) 143, **Carb Choices** 2½, **ADA Exchange** 1 fruit, 1½ milk, ½ fat

It's amazing what nutrients you can conceal in a delicious smoothie. Try adding 1 scoop each of wheat germ, unprocessed bran, and Kashi to smoothies. Add 1 serving of instant oatmeal, prepared in the microwave, to increase staying power. Two raw pasteurized eggs also add a lot of protein. Pasteurized eggs don't cause stomach or intestinal problems and are safe to eat uncooked..

Super veggie smoothies: Aside from spinach, you can add 1 scoop of protein powder or 1 cup of leftover vegetables such as lima beans, corn, or peppers, or leftover cooked rice. One cup of chopped tomatoes with 1 cup of plain yogurt and a squirt of lemon juice makes a wonderful creamy smoothie; just add 1 celery stalk and a few onion slices to the blender, and it's a fine lunch. You will find smoothies that your kids will love and want constantly—try variations.

Cut Fruit for Smoothies

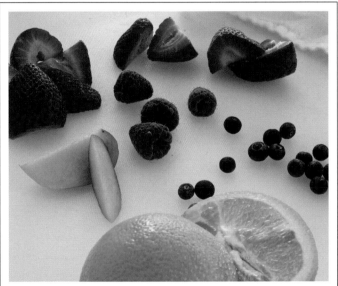

- Putting together a smoothie is a great way to use up ingredients in your fridge. Fruit in a smoothie is always a crowd favorite.

- Try using 1 cup fresh or frozen blueberries or sliced apples. Or try bananas and strawberries with sugar-free low-fat lemon yogurt.

- Cut fruit into smaller portions for a finer blend.

- For extra protein, add ½ cup more yogurt.

Adding Extra Flavor

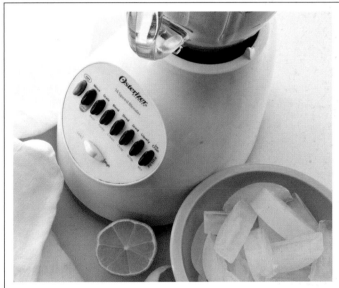

- Add even more flavor to your smoothie by mixing in extra ingredients.

- If it's that coffee or chocolate flavor you crave, blend 1 cup low-fat, sugar-free coffee yogurt with ½ cup sugar-free chocolate ice cream, ½ banana, and 2 tablespoons unprocessed bran. Be forewarned, however, that this will increase the carb content.

- Add some coffee-flavored liqueur or sugar-free chocolate syrup if you have a real chocolate craving.

STUFFED FRENCH TOAST

When cut into equal quarters, this "breakfast" makes a perfect lunch

This particular stuffing is quick and easy to make, and it can be sweet or savory. You can also add bits of fresh or dried fruit, or slices of tomato, smoked meat, or smoked salmon.

Forget about high-sugar maple syrup or other syrups; add fiber and freshness by making your own pureed fruit toppings and fruit coulis, which will contain more fiber and nutrients. You can use fresh blueberries, strawberries, raspberries,

mangos, peaches, or nectarines.

Low-fat cheese tends to melt better than fat-free cheese. If your cholesterol count is healthy, go ahead and use the low-fat cheese rather than fat-free.

Stuffed French toast is good for breakfast, lunch, or a light supper. It's totally versatile and can be made quickly with ingredients you have in your fridge. *Yield: 4 servings*

KNACK DIABETES COOKBOOK

Ingredients

For the French toast:

2 whole eggs (extra large)

2 egg whites (extra large)

$^1/_2$ cup 1 percent milk

1 teaspoon lemon zest (optional)

$^1/_2$ teaspoon Worcestershire sauce

$^1/_2$ teaspoon hot pepper sauce, more or less to taste

8 slices whole-grain bread (slightly stale is best)

4 slices low-fat, low-sodium Monterey Jack or Pepper Jack cheese (Muenster or white American cheese will also work well)

8 slices low-sodium smoked ham

For the mustard sauce:

$^1/_2$ cup low-fat mayonnaise

1 tablespoon homemade mustard

1 tablespoon minced onion

$^1/_2$ teaspoon curry powder

Calories 402, **Fat** (g) 19, **Carbohydrates** (g) 33, **Protein** (g) 26, **Fiber** (g) 4, **Saturated Fat** (g) 7, **Cholesterol** (mg) 164, **Sodium** (mg) 827, **Carb Choices** 2, **ADA Exchange** 2 starch, 3 medium-fat meat, 1 fat

Stuffed French Toast

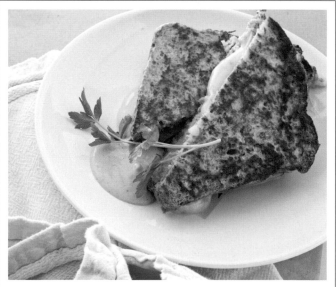

- Preheat pan over medium heat. In a large, flat-bottomed bowl, whisk eggs, milk, lemon zest, Worcestershire sauce, and hot pepper sauce.

- Place cheese and ham on four slices of bread. Close sandwiches. Dip sandwiches in egg mixture, coat-

ing both sides. Sauté until browned and cheese melts, 4 minutes per side.

- When sandwiches are done, cut them in quarters and place on a warm platter.

- Mix sauce ingredients in a bowl and serve by the teaspoonful.

French toast Is versatile: The beauty of French toast is that you can use multigrain bread. If you are trying to keep your cholesterol intake down, reduce the egg yolks, replacing each omitted yolk with another egg white. This recipe calls for using 2 yolks, but you can cut that in half. It's important to use a nonstick pan and plenty of nonstick spray (butter- or olive oil–flavored) to sauté your French toast.

French toast spreads: Make different spreads for French toast. Mix 4 heaping tablespoons low-fat ricotta cheese, 2 tablespoons Parmesan cheese, and a dash of herbs. Spread mixture onto bread and top with second slice of French toast to make a sandwich. Dip sandwich into beaten eggs and milk, and sauté. Or, mix 1 tablespoon of chopped roasted red peppers with ricotta.

Separating Egg Yolks from Whites

The Importance of Whisking

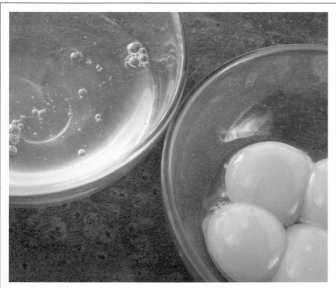

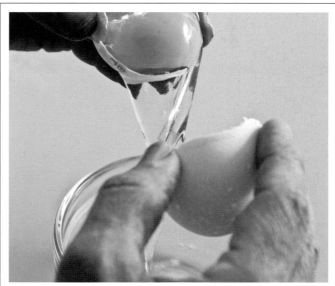

- Use a knife or the side of the bowl to split the egg.

- Have a second bowl for the yolk. After the egg is split, tip it so that the yolk sits in the small end of the shell.

- Pour the egg white into a bowl. Now slide the yolk into the other shell.

- Add the rest of the egg white to the bowl. Pour the yolk into the empty second bowl.

- It's important to whisk your eggs until emulsified. Then whisk in other ingredients.

- You can use a traditional whisk or a fork.

- You must move the utensil in a small circular motion to get every bit beaten.

- Some cooks use an immersion blender or electric eggbeater for whisking. That's a waste unless you are doing a very large amount of eggs or are working with whites that have to be beaten stiffly.

QUINOA CAKES WITH BLUEBERRIES

Quinoa with fruit is just waiting to be discovered by health-conscious cooks

Quinoa is a carbohydrate that's higher in protein than most carbohydrate foods. It will keep the family feeling full all morning with slow-release carbs, plenty of protein, and lots of fiber.

These blueberry-filled cakes are delectable and can include nuts, if desired, or you could also make a zestier version with a half cup of chopped pepperoni, ham, or roasted veggies

mixed in with the quinoa. The more you use quinoa, the more wonderful uses you'll find for it. Most health- and whole-foods stores carry quinoa. If you can't find it locally, go shopping on the Internet, and you'll have it at a great price in a day or two. Stay away from syrups for quinoa cakes; instead, dress them with a fresh fruit coulis. *Yield: 4 servings*

KNACK DIABETES COOKBOOK

Ingredients

2 extra-large eggs, beaten

2 tablespoons all-purpose flour

1 teaspoon baking powder

1 teaspoon salt

1 tablespoon lemon juice

1 teaspoon Splenda

$1/4$ teaspoon cinnamon

2 cups cooked quinoa

$1/2$ cup fresh or frozen blueberries, rinsed and dried if fresh

$1/4$ cup canola oil

Calories 507, **Fat** (g) 22, **Carbohydrates** (g) 64, **Protein** (g) 16, **Fiber** (g) 6, **Saturated Fat** (g) 3, **Cholesterol** (mg) 138, **Sodium** (mg) 787, **Carb Choices** 4, **ADA Exchange** 3 starch, 1 fruit, 1 medium-fat meat, 1 fat

Quinoa Cakes with Blueberries

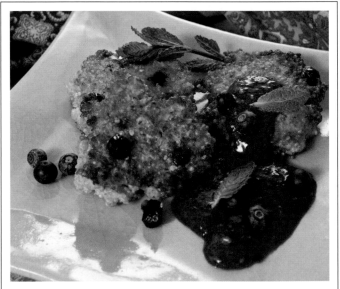

- Whisk the eggs, flour, baking powder, salt, and lemon juice together until well blended. Whisk in the Splenda and cinnamon. Fold in the quinoa and berries.

- Heat the oil in a nonstick pan over medium flame.

- Drop the batter into the oil, using about 2 tablespoons per cake.

- Let the cakes cook slowly; turn when nicely browned and hot through.

Plan ahead: Having a bowl of cooked quinoa in the refrigerator can solve a myriad of time problems such as, "What's for breakfast? Lunch? Dinner?" Just make extra when you are home on the weekend, doing some additional cooking. Use it as a base, and mix in all kinds of yummy additions. Try it with chopped turkey and dried cranberries. Or, add some leftover cold cuts and Parmesan cheese to the recipe.

Enriched meat loaf: You can also add quinoa to your favorite meatball and meat loaf recipes, substituting it for breadcrumbs. Enriched meat loaf is delicious. Add 1 cup cooked quinoa instead of bread crumbs to 1 pound ground beef or veal. Stir in ½ cup ketchup and 1 teaspoon Worcestershire sauce.

The Fine Art of Folding

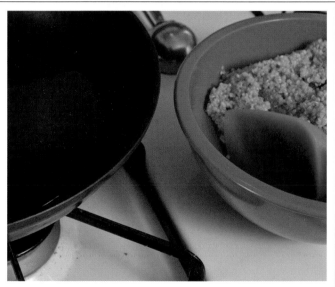

- Folding is a gentle form of mixing.

- To keep the quinoa, berries, and batter mixture from turning into mush when mixed, put it all in a big bowl.

- Then, gently and carefully turn the food over with a rubber spatula until it is mixed.

- At no point should you swoosh or roughly mix it around. This will break the berries and make the whole thing much too wet.

"Dropping" Batter

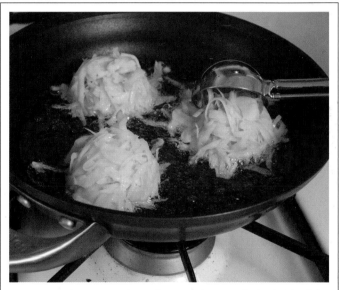

- Dropping batter into hot oil can cause a splash, which is not only messy but also potentially painful.

- For large cakes, use an ice cream scoop to place the batter into the pan. After you have carefully deposited the batter, gently push it down with the back of the scoop to flatten it out.

- Use a tablespoon for small cakes. Put one tablespoonful in the pan and place another tablespoonful on top. Then flatten it with the back of your spoon.

LIGHT LUNCH

POTATO PANCAKES WITH ONIONS
Enjoy light lunch with a wonderful crunch and taste

These delicious pancakes are quite easy to prepare. They make a nice light lunch, or you can serve them as a side with roast beef or poultry at dinner. The coarse grating gives the pancakes lots of texture and a dark golden-brown color. Be careful not to burn the oil or the pancakes. Once they start to brown, they do so quite quickly. Using a kitchen thermometer, keep the oil at 325°F to 350°F.

Do not make the batter in advance, for the potatoes will turn gray. You can, however, sauté the cakes in advance and reheat them just before serving.

Potato pancakes are traditionally served with sour cream and applesauce. They are also excellent with gravy, chutney, or fruit sauce. Leftover potato pancakes topped with salsa make good snacks. *Yield: 8 medium cakes, serves 4*

Ingredients

2 extra-large Idaho or Yukon Gold potatoes, peeled and grated

1 medium-size sweet yellow or white onion, peeled and grated

2 extra-large eggs, slightly beaten

$1/2$ cup matzo meal

1 teaspoon salt

$1/2$ teaspoon freshly ground pepper

$1/2$ cup canola oil

Calories 242, **Fat** (g) 16, **Carbohydrates** (g) 22, **Protein** (g) 4, **Fiber** (g) 3, **Saturated Fat** (g) 2, **Cholesterol** (mg) 67, **Sodium** (mg) 31, **Carb Choices** 1½, **ADA Exchange** 1½ starch, 3 fat

Potato Pancakes with Onions

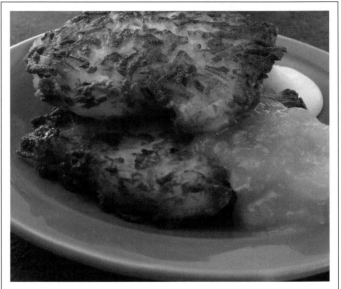

- Put the grated potato and onion in a large bowl. Whisk eggs and add to potatoes and onions; stir gently to coat.

- Stir in matzo meal, salt, and pepper. In a large frying or sauté pan, heat the canola oil over medium heat.

- Gently spoon the cakes into the hot oil. Regular size should be about ½ inch in diameter. Minis should be about 1 inch in diameter.

- Drain pancakes on paper towels or clean brown paper bags. Serve immediately.

The secret to wonderful potato pancakes—crunchy on the outside, savory on the inside—is that the potatoes are coarsely grated, not boiled and mashed. You can use a box grater and grate by hand, or the grate/shred blade on your food processor. The same blade can be used for mincing the onions. Just be sure that it all goes through and you don't have any big pieces in your batter.

Traditional spreads: Top pancakes with a spread of 4 thin slices smoked salmon, chopped, 1 tablespoon finely chopped scallions, and 1 cup low-fat, whipped cream cheese. Mash it all together; spread it on pancakes. Or, instead of applesauce, use 6 peeled and chopped fresh pears, boiled until tender with a touch of lemon juice and a dash of ground cloves. Then, mix.

Box Grater vs. Food Processor

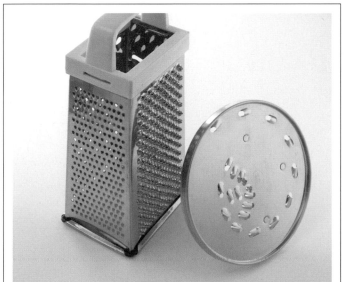

Draining Fried and Sautéed Food

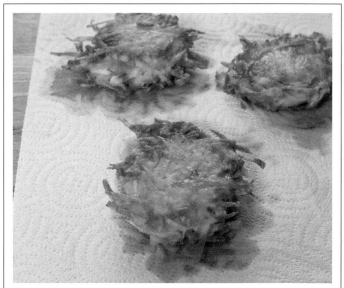

- When you use a box grater to grate potatoes, the job takes longer.

- When using a food processor, insert the grating tool. Then, cut the potatoes into long quarters so that they fit in the tubefeeder.

- Using the plastic pushing tool that comes with the food processor, push the potato quarters through the tube. As the jar fills, dump the potatoes into a bowl.

- You can use the grater or the grinding tool to mince the onions, too.

- It's important to get as much of the oil as possible off each potato pancake.

- If your frying pan is up to temperature, the food will not absorb as much oil as it would if using a pan that you did not preheat.

- Do not overload the frying pan; take pancakes out the minute they are brown.

- Place pancakes on a paper towel. Turn them in 1 minute to drain the other side.

LIGHT LUNCH

STUFFED TOASTED CHALLAH BREAD
Jewish in origin, challah is a rich, yeasty bread for the whole world to enjoy

Challah is usually made on Thursdays and sold on Fridays for nourishment over the Jewish Sabbath. One taste, and you will find it a treat no matter what your religion.

The dough is egg-based and made with yeast. A long, thick rope of dough is braided, and the bread is glazed with an egg wash to give it a rich color and high gloss.

This recipe is basically a panini, a small sandwich that is heated and pressed flat on a griddle or in a panini maker. If you do not have a panini maker, you can use a heavy pan with a brick wrapped in aluminum foil to press down on the sandwich. *Yield: 2 servings*

KNACK DIABETES COOKBOOK

Ingredients

4 thick slices challah bread

4 teaspoons low-fat mayonnaise

2 teaspoons homemade mustard (see recipe, page 208), optional

1 teaspoon dried thyme leaves

6 slices cooked turkey bacon

1 tart apple, such as Granny Smith, cored, peeled, and sliced thinly

2 teaspoons extra-virgin olive oil or nonstick olive oil-flavored spray

Calories 326, **Fat** (g) 11, **Carbohydrates** (g) 48, **Protein** (g) 8, **Fiber** (g) 1, **Saturated Fat** (g) 1, **Cholesterol** (mg) 42, **Sodium** (mg) 460, **Carb Choices** 3, **ADA Exchange** 3 starch, 2 fat

Stuffed Toasted Challah Bread

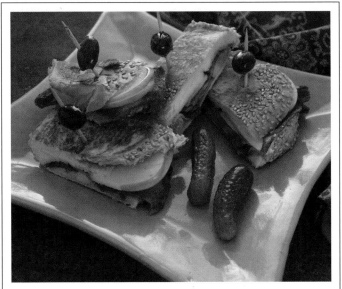

- Spread one side of each slice of bread with mayo, and mustard if desired. Sprinkle with thyme leaves.

- Arrange three slices of turkey bacon on two slices of bread; press into bread.

- Divide apple slices over bacon. Close sandwiches.

- Heat a nonstick pan over medium flame. Spray with nonstick spray or use ½ of the olive oil on the pan.

- Press sandwiches to brown sides. Turn; cook until both sides are golden. Cut into quarters; serve.

Many cooks are now buying panini makers because you can make a huge grilled sandwich and then cut it into snack-size pieces. If you get serious about your panini making, get yourself a double-sided, folding electric panini grill.

A platter full of panini made with cream cheese and salsa is wonderful for feeding a football crowd during halftime. Italian lunch places now have many variations on the panini. Get sausage or pepperoni and different cheeses with tomatoes, lettuce, and olive oil and vinegar dressing. Good old-fashioned smoked ham and Muenster cheese is another pleasing combo. Have fun and mix up!

Pressing Sandwiches

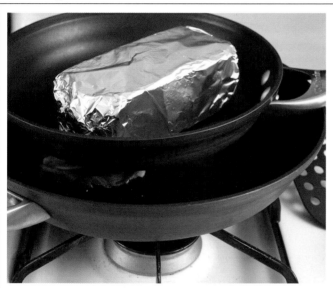

Browning Your Pressed Sandwich

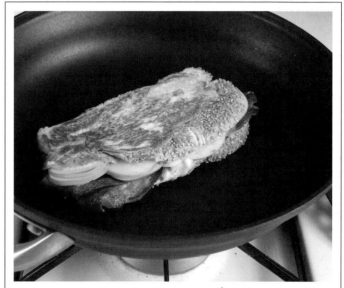

- Pressing a sandwich creates a magical transformation.

- It melds flavors, compressing them to the point of total flavor integration.

- If you don't have a panini press, improvise by using some kitchen staples. Use either the base of a heavy pan to press the sandwich, or the base of a smaller pan with a foil-wrapped brick weighing it down.

- Be sure your pans are clean inside and out prior to being used as a press.

- If you use an electric panini maker, watch your sandwiches. Bread and fillings differ enough to make frequent checking important.

- When using a frying or sauté pan on top of the stove, you will need to turn the sandwiches from time to time to check on them.

- The outside of the sandwich should be very crisp and golden brown.

- If you need to add more olive oil or nonstick spray, go ahead and use it plentifully.

ASPARAGUS SOUP, HOT OR COLD
Once you try this velvety soup, you'll want to make it again and again

This is a beautiful and elusive "green" soup that smells and tastes young and fresh. To add more color to the soup, add half a box of frozen baby peas. To make it lighter in color, substitute equal amounts of white asparagus and new potatoes for the green asparagus.

The base of the soup consists of sautéed aromatic veggies and chicken broth. Aromatic vegetables include garlic, either roasted or fresh; onions, shallots, and chives; celery, carrots, and baby turnips; and parsnips and radishes. You can also use mustard greens, fennel, kohlrabi, and celeriac (celery root).

As you adjust the ingredients to your liking, you will also adjust the taste, which makes this a tantalizing and always versatile summer soup. *Yield: 6 servings*

Ingredients

1 pound asparagus, rinsed, trimmed, and cut into 2-inch pieces

$1/4$ cup chicken broth

2 tablespoons olive oil

4 shallots, peeled and chopped coarsely

1 tablespoon plus 1 teaspoon all-purpose flour

1 cup 1 percent milk, warmed in the microwave

1 cup low-salt chicken broth, warmed in the microwave

Juice of $1/2$ lemon

$1/4$ cup dry white wine (optional)

1 teaspoon lemon zest

$1/2$ teaspoon Worcestershire sauce

Salt to taste

Freshly ground black pepper to taste

Calories 78, **Fat** (g) 4, **Carbohydrates** (g) 7, **Protein** (g) 3, **Fiber** (g) 1, **Saturated Fat** (g) 1, **Cholesterol** (mg) 4, **Sodium** (mg) 145, **Carb Choices** ½, **ADA Exchange** ½ milk, 1 fat

Asparagus Soup, Hot or Cold

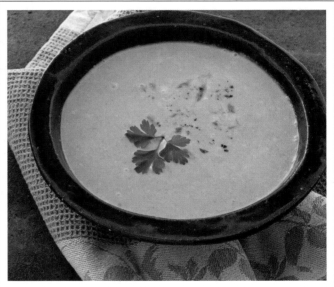

- Microwave the asparagus and chicken broth in a ceramic or glass bowl for 4 minutes. Set aside.

- Heat the olive oil at medium in a large nonstick pan; sauté the shallots.

- Stir in flour and cook 3 minutes, stirring constantly.

- Whisk in warm milk. Stir until very thick. Then whisk in broth.

- Cook soup until thickened. Whisk in the remaining ingredients. Blend the soup and asparagus until smooth.

- Cover and refrigerate. Serve well-chilled or heated.

Cream soups and cholesterol: Be wary about using real, full-fat dairy products such as whole milk, butter, sour cream, and ice cream, which are all high in saturated fat. Saturated fat raises cholesterol, while all types of fat (saturated or unsaturated) provides a lot of calories. If you choose to include some foods with saturated fat in your meals, these soups are great options. Consult your doctor to determine the best diet for you, depending on your cholesterol test readings. It's wise to make your own broth, cook your own fish and chicken, and use lots of fiber and olive oil in your diet.

Smooth Soup

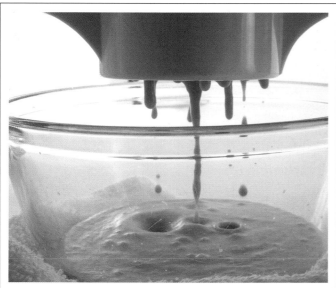

- A rough-textured soup can be rustic. However, if you want smooth soup, you need a fine blend.

- If blending doesn't get all the particles out of the soup, simply put it through a fine sieve.

- For people with digestive issues, a smooth soup is gentler on the body. The coarse texture affects the digestive system, slowing the absorption of carbohydrates.

- Keep in mind that the soup won't be completely smooth; some fiber will be there, no matter what.

Extra-Green Soup

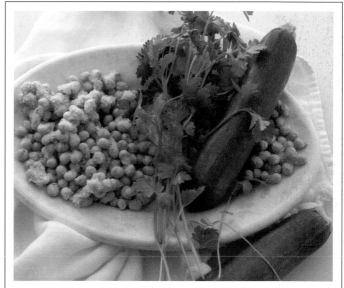

- The color of the soup will change depending on the amount of green ingredients added to it.

- To make your soup very green, add a half box of frozen peas.

- Or, add 1 sprig of chopped parsley.

- If you want added color but don't want to interfere with the flavor of the asparagus, add 1 medium-size steamed zucchini and puree with soup.

SWEDISH FRUIT SOUP

Fresh raspberries are the crown jewels of this pretty and colorful fruit soup

During the long, cold winters when fresh summer fruit was impossible to get, Scandinavians made do with dried fruits, and fruit soup was considered a dessert. Today, a cold fruit soup is an excellent summer lunch entrée.

Use dried apricots, fresh or dried peaches, or a mixture of dried fruits, as was used in the "old days." Once you start making fruit soup, you can vary it with the seasons. Melon soup, made with honeydew or cantaloupe and spiked with lime juice and ginger, is delightful. Add dried cherries or cranberries on top for a fine garnish. Garnish fruit soup with fresh mint leaves, basil leaves, toasted nuts, or fresh berries. A dollop of low-fat yogurt or sour cream is also nice. *Yield: 6 servings*

Ingredients

10–12 ounces dried apricots or peaches

¼ cup dried cherries (6–8 medium, fresh cherries)

6 cups water

1 tablespoon Splenda

1 teaspoon lemon zest

1 cinnamon stick

2 tablespoons tapioca

Juice of ½ lemon

½ teaspoon salt

1 cup fresh raspberries, rinsed

6 tablespoons low-fat sour cream or plain yogurt

Calories 78, **Fat** (g) 2, **Carbohydrates** (g) 15, **Protein** (g) 1, **Fiber** (g) 2, **Saturated Fat** (g) 1, **Cholesterol** (mg) 6, **Sodium** (mg) 7, **Carb Choice** 1, **ADA Exchange** 1 fruit

Swedish Fruit Soup

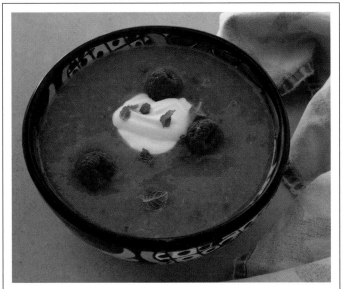

- Place the first seven ingredients in a slow cooker or double boiler, covered, on low for 2 hours. Stir occasionally.

- When the fruit is tender, stir in the lemon juice and add a pinch of salt if necessary. Remove the cinnamon stick. Chill the soup.

- At this point, you can either puree the soup or serve it chunky—it's up to you.

- Serve topped with fresh raspberries and a spoonful of low-fat sour cream or yogurt.

ZOOM

Using dried fruit: When using dried fruit, such as apricots, peaches, or a mixture of both, start cooking the soup in your slow cooker. This is a great time-saver. Dried fruits do not have to be peeled or pitted, whereas fresh ones do need more attention. Recipes that practically cook themselves are wonderful for both family and company.

• • • • RECIPE VARIATION • • • •

Fruit variety: Fruit soup can also be made with combinations of peaches and berries, such as using four blanched, pureed peaches to 1 pint fresh blueberries. For creaminess, blend in 1 cup low-fat or fat-free yogurt, and add 1 teaspoon of Tabasco sauce for spiciness. Or, try cantaloupe melon and raspberries (2 cups melon chunks to 1 pint raspberries) with 1 cup fat-free or low-fat yogurt.

Using a Double Boiler

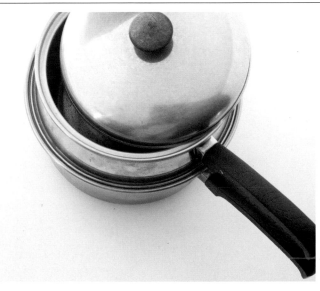

Freeze Your Soup

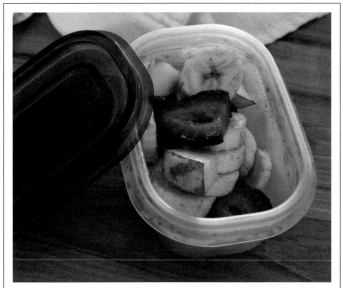

- The double boiler is wonderful for simmering sauce or soup over very low heat without burning it.

- The concept is a hot-water bath in the bottom pot and a tightly fitting top pot that sits over the boiling water.

- The boiling water should not touch the pot that sits on top.

- This is also a great way to make puddings, which easily stick to the bottom of a pan on the stove.

- Local seasonal fruits are best for making your soup. They are less traveled and freshest when in season.

- Use lots of peaches, apricots, berries, and melons—fruits in season in summer.

- Freeze the fruit for use in winter. Nothing is more

refreshing on a winter evening than to serve a fruit soup when you have a chicken or turkey roasting in the oven.

- By freezing your soups, you can now enjoy fresh "summer soups" year-round.

COLD CUCUMBER SOUP

The busy cook's dream dish is this light and luscious soup that requires no cooking

Cold cucumber soup is not cooked on the stove. It actually cooks in the acid of the lemon juice. You make it the day before, so the taste can transform from being a bit harsh to very smooth and easy on the palate.

Hot pepper sauce goes into this recipe because it adds a bit of zing. Fresh dill is far superior to dried dill, but if you can't

get the fresh stuff, by all means, use dried.

A small amount of crab or shrimp salad on top is a nice touch. Even the seafood salad you buy at the market is pretty when spooned on top. But use store-bought seafood salads sparingly because they are usually loaded with mayonnaise. *Yield: 6 servings*

Ingredients

1 English cucumber, rinsed and cut into 1-inch chunks

$1/2$ cup sweet white onions, peeled and coarsely chopped

1 quart nonfat plain yogurt

Juice of 1 fresh lemon

1 teaspoon lemon zest

2 tablespoons fresh dill weed plus sprigs for garnish, or 2 teaspoons dried dill

1 teaspoon hot pepper sauce

$1/2$ teaspoon salt, or to taste

Optional but recommended: 6 ounces crab, shrimp, or mixed seafood salad for garnishing the soup

Calories 117, **Fat** (g) 3, **Carbohydrates** (g) 15, **Protein** (g) 9, **Fiber** (g) 1, **Saturated Fat** (g) 2, **Cholesterol** (mg) 10, **Sodium** (mg) 121, **Carb Choice** 1, **ADA Exchange** 1 milk, ½ fat

Cold Cucumber Soup

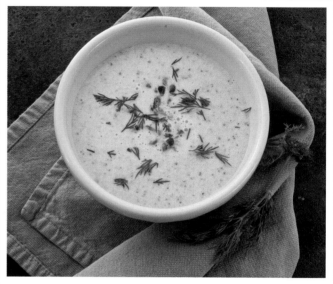

- Puree all ingredients, except for the optional salad, in a blender or food processor.

- Scrape down the sides of the blender jar from time to time, and process until very smooth.

- Chill overnight. Pour into prechilled bowls, and top with a little seafood salad, if desired.

- Add sprigs of fresh dill for flavor and decoration.

MAKE IT EASY

Make soup in advance: There is something wonderful about opening the fridge on a hot day and pulling out some icy cold soup. And this soup has just about everything you need to be cooled and well fed at the same time. Because the soup cooks in the lemon-zest acid, making it a day ahead will ensure that the soup's flavor has enough time to mellow.

ZOOM

Better ingredients mean better flavor. English "seedless" and/or "Burpee's Burp-less" cucumbers are recommended for this dish, unless you can get local, fresh ones at a roadside stand or green market. The recommended cucumbers are long and thin and unwaxed, unlike the ones in the supermarket. Use the entire cucumber after rinsing. Remember, the fresher the ingredients, the more vibrant the flavor.

Squeeze, Ream, and Zest

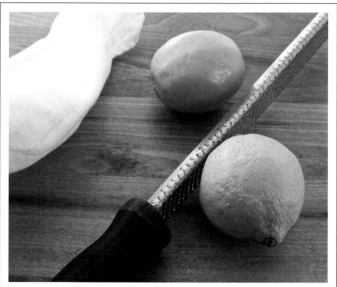

- Fresh lemons give you so much more than the reconstituted stuff in bottles. You get the zest, seeds for the kids to plant, and, of course, lovely fresh juice.

- Zest the lemon before you cut it. You can use a rasp or box grater. Rinse the lemon before zesting.

- You can use a lemon juicer to get the juice out, but a reamer works just as well.

- To make the juices flow, roll the lemon around while pressing.

Playing with Garniture

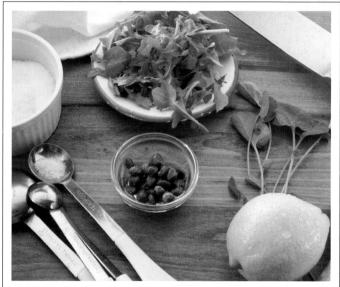

- Garniture is fun to experiment with on soups.

- Sprinkle capers or green peppercorns over the soup.

- Play with bitter greens such as arugula and watercress for an added boost of flavor. Rinse fresh herbs and

greens well in cold water, then dry on a paper towel.

- For use later, roll the greens in paper towels, put in a plastic bag, and refrigerate. They will stay crispy and bright.

COLD GARDEN TOMATO SOUP

Capturing the very essence of summer, this soup is known as gazpacho in Spain

If you buy tomatoes by the peck or bushel in August and freeze them, you can make fresh soups and sauces year-round. Nothing from a can compares with fresh.

This soup is made with some red wine and beef broth to make it a bit heartier than straight vegetable soup. But you can also make it strictly with vegetables, using vegetable broth instead of beef broth. The fun part is adding some crunchy favorites on top and then having a platter loaded with extra veggies on the side.

You can make the soup spicy or mild. Like so many soups, it's best to make it the night before and let the flavors marry in the refrigerator for a more vibrant taste. *Yield: 8 servings*

Ingredients

2 tablespoons olive oil

1 small onion, peeled and coarsely chopped

4 cloves garlic, smashed, peeled, and coarsely chopped

6 cups chopped tomatoes, fresh or canned

1 13- or 14-ounce can low-sodium beef broth

1 cup dry red wine

Juice of 1 lemon

1 teaspoon hot pepper sauce, more or less to taste

1 teaspoon Worcestershire sauce

$^1/_2$ cup each: carrots, celery, scallions, radishes, celeriac, fennel, and red and green peppers, all chopped to serve on the side with the soup

Calories 116, **Fat** (g) 4, **Carbohydrates** (g) 14, **Protein** (g) 3, **Fiber** (g) 3, **Saturated Fat** (g) 1, **Cholesterol** (mg) 0, **Sodium** (mg) 137, **Carb Choice** 1, **ADA Exchange** 3 vegetable, ½ fat

Cold Garden Tomato Soup

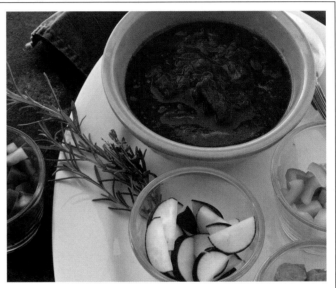

- Heat olive oil in a soup pot set over medium heat. Add onion and garlic, and sauté, stirring, until softened.

- Add tomatoes and broth. Bring to a boil and reduce heat to a simmer.

- Add wine, lemon, hot pepper sauce, and Worcester- shire sauce. Cover; simmer 15 minutes. Remove from heat and allow to cool. When cool, place in a bowl and store in the fridge.

- Either mound the chopped vegetables on a platter or lazy Susan so that people can help themselves, or add them to the soup.

MAKE IT EASY

Food processor chopping: Using the food processor as a chopper is easy and works well for onions, garlic, carrots, and other firm vegetables. It will coarsely chop tomatoes if you pulse it on and off; or, it will puree them. Cut your onions, carrots, etc., into chunks, and always pulse to get an even chop.

• • • • RECIPE VARIATION • • • •

Adding celery root or spinach: Try adding 1 cup grated celery root or 1 cup shredded fresh baby spinach to the basic recipe for Cold Garden Tomato Soup. You will also change the character of the soup by adding one fennel bulb, trimmed and shaved paper-thin.

Smash That Garlic!

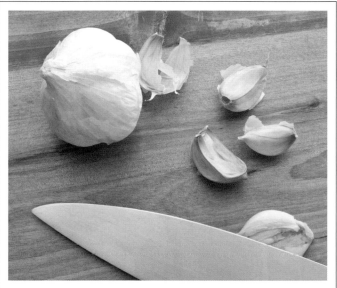

- The easiest way to prepare garlic is to smash it.

- Put the clove on a cutting board; press the flat side of a chef's knife down on the garlic and apply pressure.

- For a lot of cloves, spread them on a piece of waxed paper. Add another layer of waxed paper, then rock a heavy frying pan over the paper to smash.

- Once smashed, the garlic peels easily, and the split cloves are ready to go into the pan.

Marinating, Macerating, and Marrying Flavors

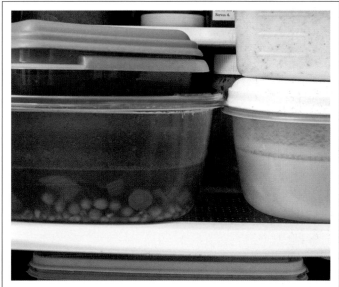

- This complex soup needs to spend time marinating so that the flavors can marry.

- When you combine flavors, they need to "cook" in order for the process of marinating or macerating to work.

- Maceration is done mostly with fruit mixed with a bit of sugar, citrus, and wine or liqueur, which becomes a sweet syrup after a period of time.

- Marinades have a special effect on meat—they tenderize it by breaking down the fibers and adding flavor.

FROSTY GREEK LEMON SOUP

Traditionally served hot, this soup can be chilled and served cold the next day

When you are in a hurry, make this everyday traditional soup and serve it hot. Put together a green salad, toast a few slices of multigrain bread, and you've got a complete meal. When you have plenty of time, make the soup in advance and then chill it for a light lunch or first course of an elegant dinner. It's light enough to be a starter and has enough protein to keep you going all afternoon if you serve it for lunch.

The wonderful thing about this soup is that you can add chopped fresh spinach, watercress, or arugula to it. Any of these make a delicious foil for the lemony flavor of the soup. However, don't use frozen spinach for this recipe; it just doesn't cut it. *Yield: 6 servings*

Ingredients

6 cups low-sodium chicken broth

Juice of 3 lemons

Salt and freshly ground black pepper to taste

3 eggs

Garnishes: $^1/_2$ cup per serving of either baby spinach, watercress or arugula; try it with $^1/_2$ cup cooked shrimp or shredded cooked chicken for extra protein.

Fresh mint leaves

Calories 91, **Fat** (g) 3, **Carbohydrates** (g) 3, **Protein** (g) 13, **Fiber** (g) 0, **Saturated Fat** (g) 1, **Cholesterol** (mg) 143, **Sodium** (mg) 695, **ADA Exchange** 1½ lean meat

Frosty Greek Lemon Soup

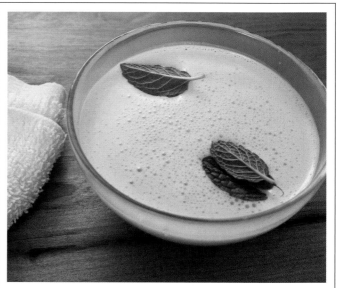

- Bring broth to a boil over high heat. Add lemon juice, salt, and pepper. Reserve one cup of hot soup. Pour soup into a large tureen or bowl for serving.

- Beat eggs in a separate bowl until pale yellow.

- When the soup has cooled slightly, whisk the reserved cup of hot soup into the egg mixture. Then, slowly whisk the mixture into the warm soup.

- Add garnishes; serve immediately, or chill for later. If chilled, give the soup a last whisk before serving, then add your garnishes.

MAKE IT EASY

Serve it how you like it: Some diners like their soup with more broth, while others like it chunky. You can get it either way with this lovely soup, depending on your whisking power. Or just serve it plain with a sprig of mint on top.

Soup as a meal: Soup makes a great lunch or supper. It's less caloric than many alternatives, such as a sandwich made with cheese and cold cuts. And, as in the case of this soup, you can toss salad greens right into it. It's also nice to add a few lightly sautéed shrimp to each bowl of soup. Chunks of cooked chicken are also an excellent addition.

Fixing Curdled Soup

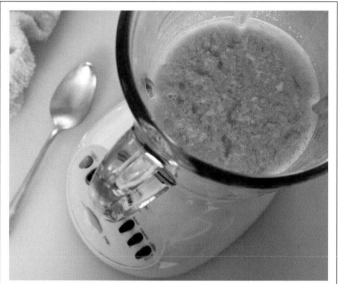

- If the egg and lemon sauce is added when the soup's too hot, it may curdle. This is unpleasant.

- However, it's simple to fix. Immediately pour the soup and 2 tablespoons of boiling water into the blender

and whirl until the curds are gone.

- Wash the bowl before returning the soup to it.

- This technique works well for curdled or lumpy custards, sauces, and soups.

Tempering

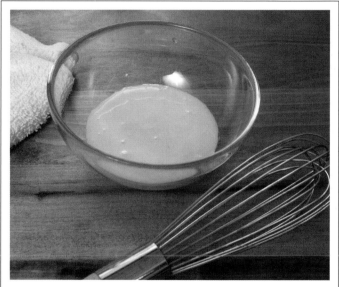

- It's important to temper ingredients that you don't want to meld and digest.

- Add a small bit of the egg or butter to the soup or sauce base. Then, slowly pour in the rest, bit by bit, stirring constantly.

- Or, you can use an electric mixer or blender rather than hand stirring.

- Your goal is to have the mixture digest itself, marrying the diverse ingredients into one smooth whole.

MEDITERRANEAN SEAFOOD SOUP

There are many recipes for seafood soup, and this is one of the healthiest

The combinations are almost endless when it comes to making seafood soup. You can make a soup base with clam broth, shrimp-shell broth, or either of these mixed with tomatoes.

The seafood combinations are all based on what's fresh in the market and your personal preferences. Mix clams and scallops, shrimp and clams, or lobster with anything you like.

Add fresh chunks of fish filet, too. A great favorite is mussels with shrimp, or use just mussels if you prefer. Mussels add a lot of broth to the base, which is a natural marriage with tomatoes. Vary the herbs used in seafood soup. Two constants are aromatic vegetables—garlic and onions sautéed in olive oil and then added to the broth. *Yield: 4 servings*

Ingredients

2 tablespoons olive oil

4 shallots, peeled and chopped

2 cloves garlic, smashed and coarsely sliced

1 quart fresh chopped tomatoes, or 1 28-ounce can crushed tomatoes

¼ cup dry red or white wine

2 pounds fresh mussels, prepared as above

1 teaspoon dried oregano

¼ cup parsley

Freshly ground black pepper

Calories 279, **Fat** (g) 12, **Carbohydrates** (g) 19, **Protein** (g) 25, **Fiber** (g) 3, **Saturated Fat** (g) 2, **Cholesterol** (mg) 54, **Sodium** (mg) 561, **Carb Choice** 1, **ADA Exchange** 1 starch, 3 lean meat

Mediterranean Seafood Soup

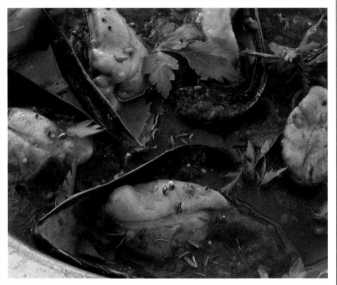

- Heat olive oil in a large pot set over medium heat. Add shallots and garlic; cook until softened. Be careful not to burn the garlic, which will then taste bitter.

- Add tomatoes, wine, and mussels; bring to a boil. As the mussels open, remove them using a slotted spoon.

- Remove the top shell from each mussel, then place them on the half shell into a soup tureen.

- Reduce heat to low; add oregano, parsley, and pepper.

- Pour the hot soup over the mussels in the tureen.

RED ● LIGHT

Mussels alive and well: Never use dead mussels or mussels that are cracked or full of mud. To ensure the safety of your mussels, find a fishmonger or retail outlet that you can trust. At home, inspect the mussels carefully. Do not leave them in a plastic bag—lack of air will kill them. Discard any that are cracked, won't close, or are wide open. Rinse under cool running water, then tap two together. Find two that make a sharp click when hit, and use one as your control. If you get a hollow sound, the mussel is dead or slightly open. Set it aside; if it doesn't "sound" right, discard.

Cleaning Mussels

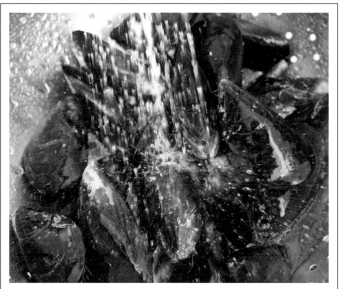

- Mussels from the market are farm raised. However, if you live on a rocky coastline with mussels thriving in clean water, you can gather them yourself. Check with your local health department.

- Farm-raised mussels are clean. They have no sand, and are "beardless."

- If you get wild mussels, soak them for 2 hours in fresh water with ½ cup of cornmeal. Mussels will pump it through their systems, expelling the sand.

- Pull off the beards (the curly threads that help the mussel cling to the rocks), and they're ready to use.

Tomatoes for Mediterranean Soup

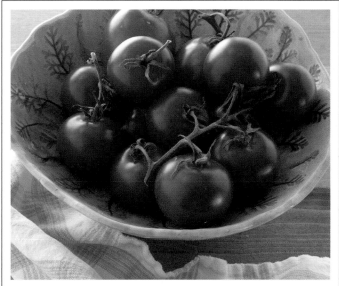

- For this recipe, you can use a variety of tomatoes, either fresh or frozen. You can find really good ones in cans and boxes.

- The best are imported from Italy and come in a box. They provide fresh flavor to your homemade variety.

- If you're using fresh, rinse a pound of ripe plum tomatoes or cherry tomatoes, remove the stem ends, and blend them.

- Strain to remove seeds and pulp.

ITALIAN SAUSAGE & BEAN SOUP

This soup combines flavors that work together and marry well

You can prepare this soup anytime because zucchini is available year-round. The zucchini should not go into the soup at the outset because it will get mushy, so we recommend adding it toward the end of the cooking process.

Soak the dry beans overnight, then cook them for 3 hours or until tender. You can use canned beans, but always drain and rinse them before adding to the soup.

Italian sausage is either hot or sweet, and either can be used in this recipe. If you are feeding young children, you probably don't want anything too hot. A good sausage will have a nice amount of fennel in it, which imparts a luscious flavor. This recipe is best used in moderation with the rest of your diet.
Yield: 8 servings

Ingredients

2 pounds Italian-style turkey sausage, in links, cut into chunks

¹/₂ cup water

2 tablespoons olive oil, if needed

1 cup sweet onions, red or white, peeled and chopped

4 cloves garlic, smashed and peeled

2 quarts chicken broth

¹/₂ package (16-ounce) dry white beans, soaked overnight, or 2 13-ounce cans cannellini beans, drained and rinsed

4 medium-size zucchini, ends removed, cut in half lengthwise and into 1-inch chunks

1 tablespoon dried rosemary or 3 tablespoons fresh rosemary

1 tablespoon dried oregano or 2 tablespoons fresh oregano

¹/₄ cup chopped fresh parsley

Salt and freshly ground black pepper to taste

Calories 438, **Fat** (g) 22, **Carbohydrates** (g) 37, **Protein** (g) 26, **Fiber** (g) 8, **Saturated Fat** (g) 7, **Cholesterol** (mg) 37, **Sodium** (mg) 1345, **Carb Choices** 2, **ADA Exchange** 2 starch, 1 vegetable, 3 medium-fat meat, 1 fat

Italian Sausage & Bean Soup

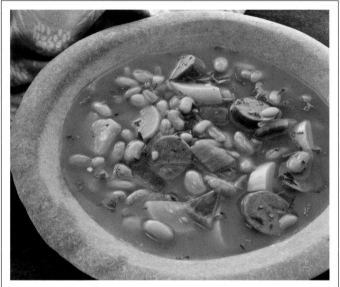

- Place sausage in a soup pot with water. Bring to a boil; cook, turning occasionally until water is gone and sausages are firm to the touch. Drain on paper towels.

- Reduce heat to low. If pot is dry, add olive oil. Sauté onions and garlic until tender. Add broth and beans.

Slice sausage links into bite-size chunks and add them to soup pot.

- Cook 30 minutes. Add the rest of the ingredients and simmer, covered, 30 minutes more or until the beans are tender. Dried, soaked beans will take longer than canned beans.

• • • • RECIPE VARIATION • • • •

Herbs in soup: Add various dried herbs to this or any soup, but fresh herbs should be added near the end of the cooking process. Keep in mind that, when cooked too long, herbs lose flavor. Start with a few, and add more when soup is closer to being done. Rosemary, oregano, and basil are used in Italian cooking. Fennel seeds and bulbs sliced thinly are tasty additions, as are the top greens.

Vegetable substitutions: An alternative to zucchini is the same quantity of yellow summer squash. It has a slightly buttery flavor. Put it in toward the end of the cooking process. Add in green beans or grated carrots, which add a nice color boost. For a subtle change in flavor, substitute chicken broth for vegetable, beef, or turkey broth. Chopped parsley and chives are delicious garnishes.

Cooking Italian Sausage

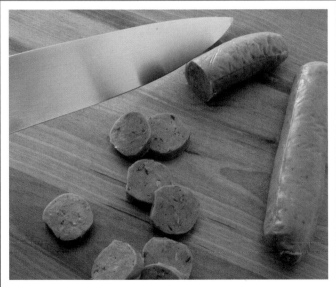

- When you make soup, use link sausage. Bulk sausage just turns into ground meat.

- The links cut nicely into bite-size rounds.

- After you've started the sausage in water and it begins to plump, prick it with a fork so that any fat runs out.

- Some turkey sausage is so lean that you may need a bit of olive oil. If there is some fat in the sausage, drain the fat before returning the sausage to the pan.

Cutting Summer Squash

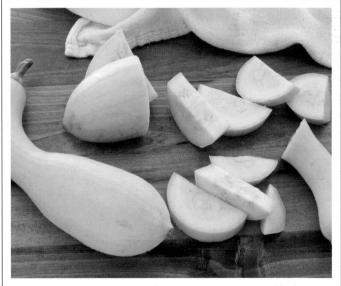

- Summer squash is quite bland but very pretty.

- You can cut in various ways to make your soup more attractive.

- Try cutting it in julienne strips, which cook almost instantly. Cutting it crosswise in coins is very easy and attractive.

- Half-coins are also very pretty and easy. Simply cut the squash lengthwise and then, holding it together, cut it crosswise.

PUMPKIN SOUP WITH ALMONDS

The almonds are toasted and used as a topping for this festive soup

Fresh pumpkins are a delicious food source. Sugar pumpkins are very sweet and are great for pies and soups, and as a side vegetable. Larger jack-o-lantern pumpkins are not as sweet but are a good source of food.

Although the recipe below calls for a garnish of toasted almonds, you can use toasted walnuts, pecans, peanuts, or hazelnuts for variety. Just be sure to toast them first.

Finely sliced jicama or chopped tart apple sprinkled over the hot soup adds a nice, crunchy contrast. The most interesting dishes feature contrasts in both flavor and texture—sweet and tart, soft and crunchy. *Yield: 6 servings*

Ingredients

2 tablespoons low-fat margarine, or canola or olive oil

2 medium-size onions, peeled and finely chopped

2 13-ounce cans pumpkin puree, unsweetened and unspiced, or 4 cups freshly roasted pumpkin, pureed

1/4 teaspoon ground nutmeg

Juice of 1 fresh lemon

1 teaspoon grated lemon zest

4 cups chicken broth

Hot pepper sauce to taste

Salt to taste

1/2 cup medium cream (optional)

Garnish: 1 cup slivered almonds, toasted

Calories 244, **Fat** (g) 5, **Carbohydrates** (g) 50, **Protein** (g) 4, **Fiber** (g) 15, **Saturated Fat** (g) 1, **Cholesterol** (mg) 0, **Sodium** (mg) 743, **Carb Choices** 3, **ADA Exchange** 2 starch, 1 fruit, 1 fat

Pumpkin Soup with Almonds

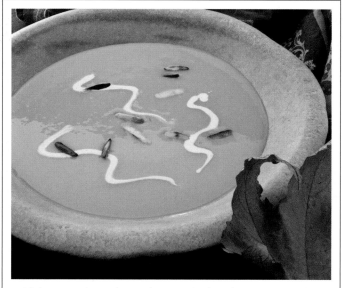

- Melt margarine or heat oil in a large soup pot over medium heat.

- Sauté onions until softened, about 4 to 5 minutes. Slowly whisk in all the remaining ingredients, minus the cream and almonds.

- Reduce heat, cover, and simmer 15 minutes. Just before serving, whisk in the cream, if desired.

- Toast almonds under the broiler. Serve the soup in prewarmed bowls; sprinkle the almonds on top just before serving.

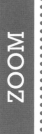

A fresh pumpkin is best used roasted, either in the oven wrapped in foil, or in the microwave wrapped in wax or freezer paper. Some supermarkets sell fresh pumpkins peeled and ready to bake or boil. If you roast your pumpkin, cut it in half and scrape the seeds out. However, if time is of the essence, open a couple of cans of pumpkin. Be sure that it's plain, not sweetened and not spiced for pie.

Butternut squash soup with almonds: The flavors in pumpkin and butternut squash are similar, so you can substitute butternut squash for pumpkin (2 13-ounce cans, or 4 cups fresh). Using butternut squash will provide less carbohydrate. Butternut squash can often be found in supermarkets already peeled and ready to bake or boil.

Working with Fresh Pumpkin

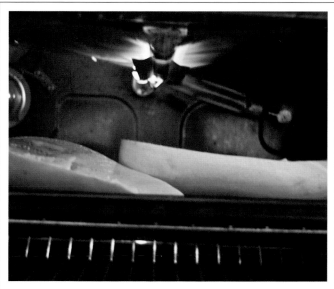

- Some cooks insist that you first peel and cube a fresh pumpkin, and then boil it to soften it.

- After you boil the pumpkin, drain it in a colander to get the moisture out before roasting.

- If your pumpkin is peeled and cut up, simply put it in a roasting pan with 1 cup of water in the bottom and roast it, covered with aluminum foil, at 300°F until fork-tender.

- If unpeeled, cut it in half and roast it in a pan with 1 cup of water until it's fork tender. Then scoop out the meat.

Roasting Almonds

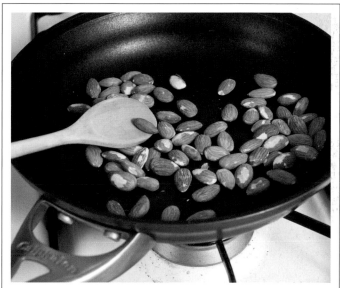

- You can roast almonds either in a pan on top of the stove or under the broiler.

- You must watch them carefully so they don't burn, and shake the pan often to turn them.

- Slivered almonds are really good as garniture and cheaper than whole ones, which you'd then have to chop.

- The same is true of walnut and pecan pieces.

MUSHROOM VEGETABLE SOUP

Wheat berries make this a very hearty soup that requires a little patience from the cook

For this recipe, it's important to precook the wheat berries for 2 to 3 hours. If you don't have time, substitute the berries with 1 cup of cooked wild rice, brown rice, or quinoa.

Using a mixture of mushrooms enriches this soup. It seems that the darker the mushrooms, the more flavorful they are. White mushrooms are the least tasty in soup. If you have an

Asian market handy, buy dried black mushrooms. Soak them according to package directions and add to your soup for a particularly rich flavor. Fresh chopped sage leaves are an excellent herb for this soup. Of course, you can use thyme or rosemary; however, fresh parsley is almost always the herb of choice to add as a garnish. *Yield: 6 servings*

Ingredients

¹/₄ cup olive oil

2 medium-size onions, peeled and chopped

4 garlic cloves, smashed, peeled, and chopped

2 carrots, peeled and shredded

1 cup frozen baby peas

1 cup chopped fresh tomatoes (skin on is fine)

1 cup cooked wheat berries, wild rice, quinoa, or brown rice

6 cups beef broth

¹/₂ cup dry red wine

2 tablespoons olive oil

4 cups fresh mushrooms, different varieties

5 fresh sage leaves, shredded

Calories 266, **Fat** (g) 15, **Carbohydrates** (g) 23, **Protein** (g) 8, **Fiber** (g) 4, **Saturated Fat** (g) 2, **Cholesterol** (mg) 0, **Sodium** (mg) 28, **Carb Choice** 1, **ADA Exchange** 1 starch, 1 vegetable

Mushroom Vegetable Soup

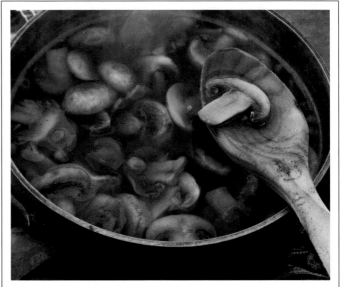

- Heat ¼ cup olive oil in a large soup pot over medium heat. Add onions and garlic. Stir frequently.

- When onions and garlic are softened, add carrots, peas, tomatoes, wheat berries, broth, and wine.

- Cover and cook over low heat for 30 minutes. While the soup is cooking, heat 2 tablespoons olive oil and sauté mushrooms in a separate pan.

- Add mushrooms and sage to soup pot, bring to a boil, and serve hot.

More on mushrooms: Mushrooms may taste meaty, but they offer very little protein. They have an earthy quality that marries well with other flavors. Exotic mushrooms, such as chanterelles and morels, have distinctive flavors and are very expensive. If you can find them, hens-of-the-woods are absolutely delicious. Shiitake mushrooms are delicate and rich-flavored. Mushrooms also absorb the flavors of the aromatic vegetables, herbs, and gravies that surround them in any dish. If you want pure, unadulterated mushroom flavor, sauté them in olive oil.

Gathering and Cleaning Mushrooms

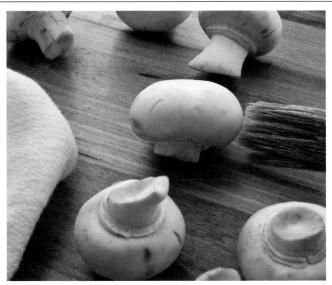

- Mushrooms should first be brushed clean or wiped with a paper towel.

- Mushrooms are commercially grown in horse manure. Before use, the manure is treated with thermophyllic bacteria, which is then burned away, purifying the manure.

- If you collect wild mushrooms, go with an expert mycologist, who can direct you to the safe ones.

- Remember that for every safe mushroom, there is a poisonous one that looks similar. To be safe, buy your mushrooms at the supermarket.

Cooking Wheat Berries and Wild Rice

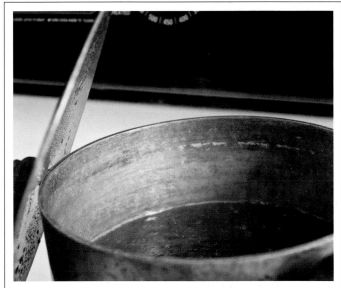

- Wheat berries and wild rice require a good deal of cooking time.

- Wheat berries must simmer for 3 hours over low heat, covered. They are done when they are chewable.

- Wild rice needs to simmer for 60 to 100 minutes.

- Wild rice morphs from little brown spikes into "blooms" when done. The kernel grows, softens, and pops the hulls apart.

IRISH LEEK & POTATO SOUP

Low-fat milk replaces the cream in this classic dish with pleasing results

The Irish are famous for their dairy products as well as potatoes and green foods, such as leeks. All those ingredients come together here to make a classic soup, but this one is lower in fat.

The traditional version of this recipe calls for both leeks and onions. You'll find that the flavor is more delicate when only leeks are used. If you'd like to include onions, use the Vidalia variety, which is grown in Vidalia, Georgia, and has a fine, sweet flavor. You can use any baking potato in this soup, including russets, New England, Maine, Yukon Gold, and Idaho potatoes. Do not use new potatoes because they are too waxy and can become sticky. *Yield: 6 servings*

KNACK DIABETES COOKBOOK

Ingredients

4 large baking potatoes, peeled and cut into chunks

1 quart chicken broth

$1/4$ cup low-fat margarine

6 leeks, white parts, cleaned and chopped

3 tablespoons all-purpose flour

Warm broth from cooking the potatoes

2 cups low-fat milk, warmed in the microwave

Salt and freshly ground pepper to taste

Calories 304, **Fat** (g) 2, **Carbohydrates** (g) 62, **Protein** (g) 11, **Fiber** (g) 6, **Saturated Fat** (g) 1, **Cholesterol** (mg) 4, **Sodium** (mg) 494, **Carb Choices** 4, **ADA Exchange** 4 starch

Irish Leek & Potato Soup

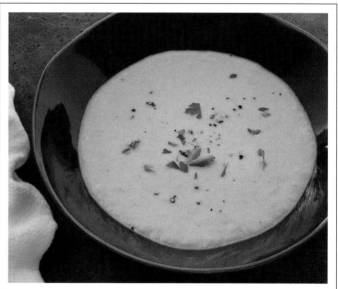

- Put potatoes in a large soup pot with chicken broth. Bring to a boil; reduce heat to a simmer. Cover and cook until potatoes are tender, about 20 minutes.

- Melt margarine over medium heat in a separate pot. Add leeks. When leeks are soft, add flour; mix well.

- Drain potatoes, saving the broth in which they were cooked. Whisk the warm broth into the leek and flour mixture and then whisk in the warm milk.

- Take time to mash potatoes with a potato masher or ricer.

78

MAKE IT EASY

For the recipe below, choose any good baking potato. Then mash it using an eggbeater or potato masher. Many cooks and chefs use a gadget called a "ricer" to mince the potato. You basically press a cooked potato through holes in the ricer. This makes perfect rice-shaped potatoes ready for the soup.

ZOOM

More on potatoes: Potatoes are one of the most interesting tubers. New potato varieties, with the exception of the finger-shaped fingerling, are round and small. The thin skin can be either yellow, brown, purple, or red. New potatoes that are a rich shade of purple can be added to mashed potatoes for extra color. These potatoes taste exactly like the brown-, yellow-, and red-skinned varieties.

A Good, Sharp Peeler

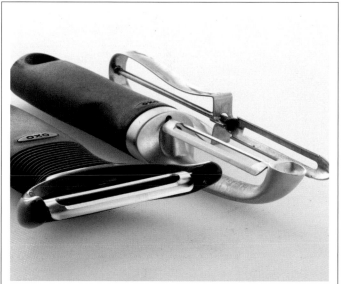

Exciting Potato Starch

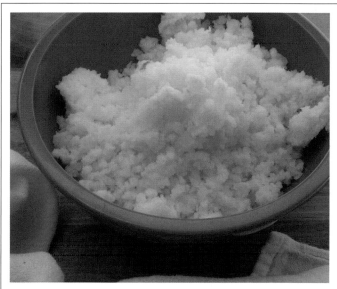

- A sharp vegetable peeler is an essential, invaluable tool. It will save you time and frustration, and it will save you food.

- If you use a knife to peel, even a very sharp one, you will waste quite a bit of potato.

- When your peeler gets dull, throw it out. It should be comfortable to hold with a firm grip.

- When you find one you like, buy extras. Then your family and friends can help with the peeling.

- Have you ever made gummy or pasty mashed potatoes? This is the result of the starch in the potatoes getting "excited" and changing its nature.

- Those shy potatoes must be mashed carefully. If you blend or process potatoes for use in soup, the starch will get gummy, with the consistency of library paste.

- Handling your potato starch carefully will prevent it from turning to a gummy mess.

TURKEY MEATBALL SOUP

A healthy version of the classic Italian wedding soup, complete with tiny meatballs

Spicy little meatballs, made with ground turkey instead of beef, are a perfect addition to many nutritious soups. This recipe, a variation on Italian wedding soup, which contains pasta and meatballs made from beef, offers reduced amounts of fat and cholesterol. Tiny pearl onions are lovely in this soup. You can buy them peeled and frozen to save time and effort.

The more veggies you add, the better the soup. Add a can of cannellini beans and some extra broth to stretch the soup.

Plenty of herbs are another essential addition. Use rosemary, oregano, and/or sage. Always sprinkle snipped chives and chopped parsley on top. Another masterful touch is a sprinkle of Italian hot pepper flakes. *Yield: 8 servings*

Ingredients

For the meatballs:

1 pound ground turkey

2 eggs, beaten

$^1/_4$ cup chili sauce

1 teaspoon Worcestershire sauce

$^1/_2$ cup bread crumbs

$^1/_2$ cup finely grated Parmesan cheese

1 teaspoon each: dried oregano, fennel seeds

Salt and pepper, to taste

For the soup:

$^1/_4$ cup olive or canola oil

24 tiny pearl onions

4 cloves garlic, smashed, peeled, and sliced

3 medium-size yellow onions, peeled and chopped

1 bag (8 ounces) prepared baby carrots

$^1/_2$ pound fresh green string beans, trimmed and cut into 1-inch pieces

1 $^1/_2$ quarts low-sodium chicken broth

1 28-ounce can crushed Italian tomatoes

2 teaspoons dried oregano or 2 tablespoons fresh oregano

1 bay leaf

$^1/_2$ teaspoon fennel seeds

Calories 250, **Fat** (g) 13, **Carbohydrates** (g) 18, **Protein** (g) 17, **Fiber** (g) 3, **Saturated Fat** (g) 3, **Cholesterol** (mg) 34, **Sodium** (mg) 775, **Carb Choice** 1, **ADA Exchange** 3 vegetable, 2 medium-fat meat

Turkey Meatball Soup

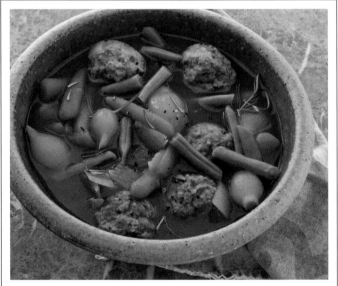

- Preheat oven to 350°F. Cover a cookie sheet with aluminum foil and spray with nonstick spray.

- Thoroughly mix all of the meatball ingredients. Form small meatballs; place on cookie sheet. Bake 20 to 30 minutes. Drain meatballs on paper towel; cool.

- Heat oil in a pot over medium heat. Add pearl onions, garlic, and chopped onions; sauté until soft.

- Stir in remaining ingredients, one at a time. Bring soup to a boil, and cook until carrots are tender. Add meatballs.

• • • • RECIPE VARIATION • • • •

The meat in your meatballs: Turkey is recommended for this recipe; however, you can use an equivalent amount of lean ground beef. The turkey is lower in calories than the beef. A mixture of beef, veal, and pork, called the meat loaf mix and available in your grocery store's meat department, is classic for meat loaf and makes a very tasty meatball. However, if you are concerned about reducing fat, cholesterol, and your caloric intake, use the turkey with the spices and herbs recommended in this recipe. Plus, if you bake the meatballs as opposed to frying them, and then drain them on paper towels, you'll eliminate much of the fat.

How to Make Meatballs

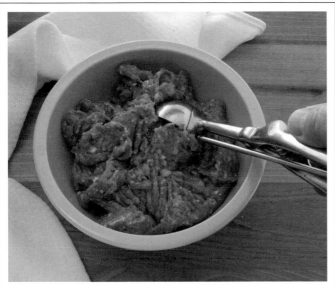

- For tiny meatballs, use a small measuring spoon to scoop up the meat mixture. For extra-tiny ones, use a melon baller.

- When making large meatballs for spaghetti sauce, use a small ice-cream scoop.

- Roll the meatballs around between your palms to compress so they don't fall apart.

- If your meatballs are all the same size, they will cook at the same rate if your oven temperature is even from front to back.

Frying vs. Baking Meatballs

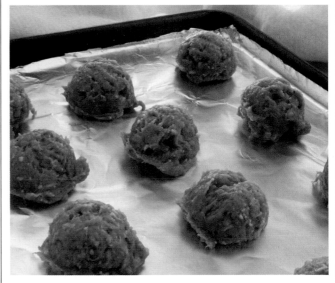

- For years cooks fried meatballs in deep fat, using lots of oil, and there is a slight advantage to that method.

- The outside of the meatball will sear, and the inside will stay moister than when baked.

- However, baking does not require the constant attention that frying does.

- By the time you add them to a pot of soup or pasta sauce, the meatballs will come out pretty much the same. Just be sure to season them well.

HOMEMADE BROTH

Homemade broth is a great way to save money, and it's naturally low in sodium

When making homemade broth, the basic techniques differ slightly depending on whether you use meat or poultry.

The classic broth, and probably the easiest, is that made from leftover Thanksgiving turkey for turkey soup. It's also easy to make chicken broth from the remains of a large roasted chicken. Or you can pick up a few pounds of chicken necks and backs at the supermarket. They make wonderful stock and lots of it. Just add aromatic vegetables and herbs.

If you have a friendly butcher who will save you some meaty beef bones, you're lucky. Otherwise you can buy short ribs or oxtails for beef stock. Or, if you've done a large standing rib roast, you have the basis for excellent beef stock. *Yield: 2 quarts*

Ingredients

4-5 pounds chicken necks and backs, or beef bones such as oxtails, neck bones, or short ribs

Water, enough to cover the bones

1 carrot, cut into chunks

2 stalks celery, cut in 1-inch chunks

Sea salt to taste

1 teaspoon Worcestershire sauce

Free Diabetes Exchange

Homemade Broth

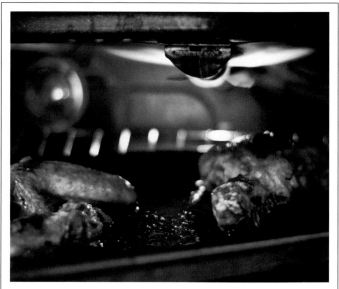

- Place bones (or necks and backs) in an ovenproof roasting pan. Broil until brown. Turn; brown other side.

- Place browned bones in a stockpot. Deglaze the roasting pan with enough water to dissolve and scrape bits off the bottom; add scrapings to stockpot.

- Add remaining ingredients to stockpot and bring to a boil on stove. Reduce heat to a simmer, cover, and cook 2 to 3 hours.

- Cool broth and skim off any fat. Remove bones. Strain; freeze for future use.

Stocking your freezer with broth: You can freeze stock in ice cube trays for use in sauces, or in 1-cup containers, or by the quart. After you've frozen a couple of ice cube trays' worth, place the cubes in plastic ziplock bags. Then, when making sauces, add the cubes as you need them. Try to keep a couple of quarts of chicken stock and beef stock in your freezer for making quick soup. You will then just need a few vegetables, any leftover meat, and some pasta or rice. You can actually make a lunch of leftovers added to stock. And, if you need more sustenance, just quick-thaw and cut up a frozen boneless chicken breast and toss it in the soup.

Why Brown the Bones?

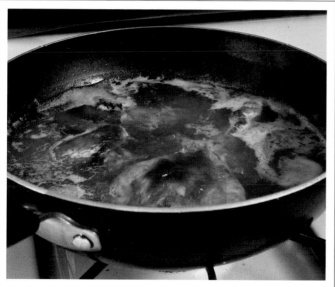

- When you brown the bones for stock, it creates a nice, rich color.

- You will also get "fonds": the meat essences—the brown bits on the bottom of the pan, concentrated nuggets of flavor.

- These nuggets mix into the broth when water is added.

- They should be scraped up with a wooden spoon as the warm water is added. Then add them to your broth for a rich flavor.

Broth vs. Stock

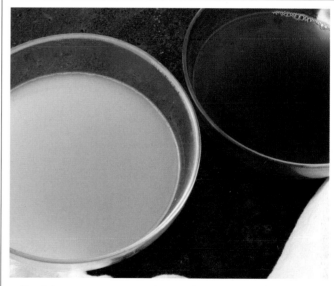

- Stock is more concentrated than broth. It's much richer and stronger, and is necessary for good sauces.

- Concentrate your broth by reducing it in volume, cooking it down at high heat, uncovered.

- Or you can tip the top of the pot and continue to cook your broth until it's richly reduced.

- You can add red wine to beef stock and white wine to poultry stock. Bones from roasting a duck or chicken make a truly delicious stock for soup.

CURRIED CHICKEN SALAD

Served with rice and grapes, this salad makes a great summer lunch

Curry is a marvelous combination of spices. It enhances meat, poultry, seafood, eggs, and vegetables. It can be whisked into salad dressings, mixed with mayonnaise, whirled into gravies and sauces—curry goes with just about everything.

The trick is to buy a mild curry powder and then make it as hot as you like with cayenne pepper. It's even an excellent condiment when mixed with mustard and then added to mayonnaise to be served with cold meats.

Many people find curry quite entrancing, but for first-timers, it's wise not to overdo it. *Yield: 4 servings*

Ingredients

For the dressing:

1 egg substitute

Juice of 1 lemon

2 teaspoons curry powder, or to taste

Pinch of salt

Few drops hot pepper sauce

$^1/_4$ cup extra-virgin olive oil

For the salad:

2 tablespoons olive oil

1 pound boneless, skinless chicken breasts

$^1/_4$ cup dry white wine

2 cups cooked rice (basmati or arborio)

1 cup green or red grapes, halved

$^1/_2$ cup roasted peanuts, almonds, or walnuts, low-sodium or salt-free

Salad greens, enough for **4** generous servings

Sliced avocado for garnish (optional)

Calories 525, **Fat** (g) 28, **Carbohydrates** (g) 34, **Protein** (g) 31, **Fiber** (g) 2, **Saturated Fat** (g) 4, **Cholesterol** (mg) 110, **Sodium** (mg) 85, **Carb Choices** 2, **ADA Exchange** 1 starch, 1 fruit, 4 medium-fat meat, 2 fat

Curried Chicken Salad

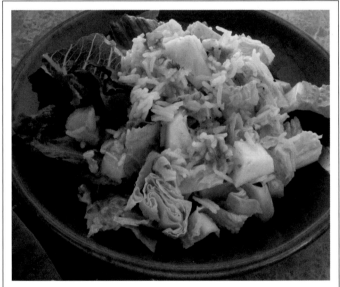

- To make dressing, blend all but olive oil in a blender. Slowly add oil, a few drops at a time. Set aside.

- Pour oil into a nonstick sauté pan set over medium heat. Add chicken; brown on both sides.

- Pour in wine, reduce heat.

- Simmer until chicken is done, 8 to 10 minutes, depending on thickness.

- Slice chicken. Add chicken/wine liquid to rice in bowl. Combine all ingredients minus salad greens in bowl. Stir in dressing; serve over greens and garnish with avocado.

Garnishes and substitutions: Although this recipe calls for whisking curry powder and hot pepper sauce into an oil-based dressing, you can also mix it with a base of low-fat mayonnaise, substituting the mayo for oil. Vary the fruit used in this recipe. Green grapes and melon balls are quite lovely; however, pineapple is excellent, and honeydew balls are also very nice. Be careful to eat fruit in moderation and follow your specific diet. Peanuts, toasted walnuts, and other varieties of nuts are great garnishes for curried dishes.

Make your own chutney: Mango chutney is particularly good with curried chicken, shrimp, or any cold meat. Combine 1 ripe mango, 1 teaspoon fresh ginger, the juice of half a lime, and 1 teaspoon hot sauce. Mash it all together with a fork, and you have chutney.

Chicken for Salad

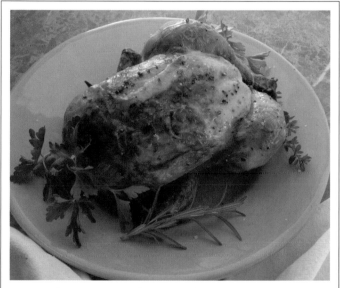

Removing the Avocado Pit

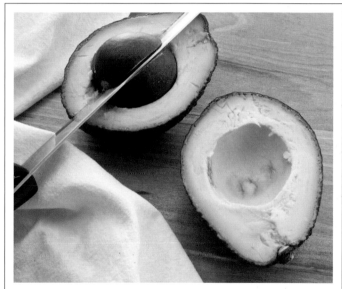

- As an alternative to cooking the chicken, use last night's leftover roast chicken or rotisserie chicken from the supermarket.

- These supermarket chickens are easy on the home cook but often are dried out, tough, and tasteless.

- To avoid this, try to get one just as it comes off the spit.

- Save money by using one roast chicken for several different meals.

- Your final meal from this bird could be a rich chicken soup.

- To remove the pit, cut the avocado in half and twist it. One side will hold the pit.

- To get the pit out without mashing the avocado, place it on a cutting board, pit side up. Using a sharp chef's knife, carefully hit the pit.

- The knife should go partway into the hard pit and hold. Then, just pull the pit out with the knife.

- If holding the avocado while removing the pit, be careful not to stab through the avocado and into your hand.

ORANGE-GLAZED CHICKEN SALAD

This lovely salad has a tropical aroma and goes well with fresh, spicy arugula

For this meal, you can use boneless, skinless chicken breasts or, for a bit more flavor, thighs. Either way, a glaze is a delicious way to enhance the chicken.

Some of the more luscious garnishes for this salad include sliced water chestnuts, mandarin oranges, toasted nuts, or all of the above. You will also find that a bed of cold wild rice sets off the chicken and arugula perfectly. This salad is great for people with diabetes; although it does have a sweet flavor, the jam is sugar free and the orange juice is freshly squeezed. Brown or wild rice is a high-quality complex carbohydrate that slows the digestive process. The protein from chicken adds staying power to the meal. *Yield: 4 servings*

Ingredients

$^1/_2$ cup sugar-free orange marmalade

2 tablespoons light soy sauce

Juice of $^1/_2$ orange, freshly squeezed

1 teaspoon freshly grated gingerroot

$^1/_2$ teaspoon red pepper flakes, or to taste

1 pound boneless, skinless chicken breasts or thighs

2 cups arugula or other greens

$^1/_2$ cup citrus dressing or vinaigrette

1 cup cooked wild or brown rice (optional)

Optional garnishes: dried cranberries; toasted pine nuts; water chestnuts, drained and rinsed; mandarin oranges, drained and rinsed

Calories 305, **Fat** (g) 8, **Carbohydrates** (g) 15, **Protein** (g) 30, **Fiber** (g) 1, **Saturated Fat** (g) 2, **Cholesterol** (mg) 82, **Sodium** (mg) 395, **Carb Choice** 1, **ADA Exchange** 1 fruit, 4 very lean meat

Orange-Glazed Chicken Salad

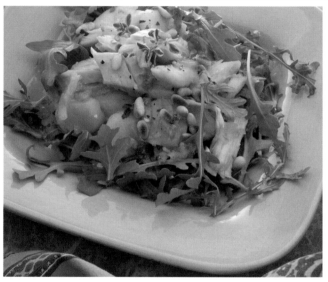

- Preheat broiler to 350°F; set rack 8 to 10 inches from heat source. Mix first five ingredients together in a small bowl; warm in microwave for 90 seconds or until marmalade is melted.

- Place chicken on nonstick sprayed pan; coat with orange glaze. Broil 5 minutes per side, being careful not to burn it. Turn; brush glaze on second side and broil another 5 minutes.

- Cut chicken into strips; arrange greens on platter. Pour dressing over greens. Mix rice with chicken. Spoon chicken over greens; garnish as desired.

Various glazes: You can also glaze chicken with fresh raspberries mixed with sugar-free raspberry jam. Or, make a very nice cranberry glaze by reducing cranberry juice and adding dried cranberries. The glaze will also drizzle into and add flavor to the salad dressing. You can mix extra reduced juice with the dressing, or add it to room-temperature brown or wild rice to give your salad body. Finally, you can easily mix glazes such as cranberry and orange, or prune and orange. All are very good. Switching the greens: The fresher and crisper the greens, the better. Arugula is called for here, but you can use mixed field greens, baby spinach, or romaine.

The Slow Broil

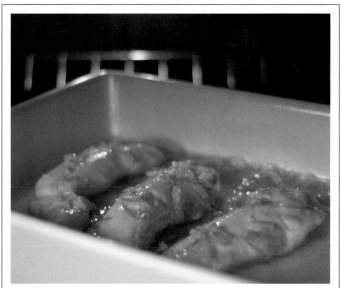

- Slow-broiling glazed meat or poultry has some advantages, the first being that it prevents the outside from burning while leaving the inside done.

- You do not want to see any pink meat in poultry.

- You can get slow-broil results on a charcoal grill by banking the coals after they turn white and placing the chicken away from the direct heat.

- Be sure to cover the grill so that the inside of the chicken cooks thoroughly.

Alternative to Broiling

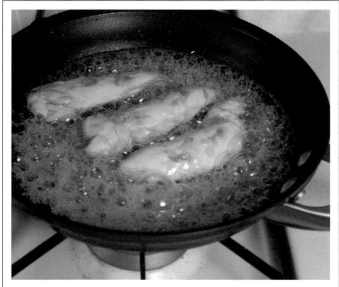

- As an alternative to broiling, poach the chicken in the glaze used in this recipe.

- Bring the glaze to a simmer in a pan on top of the stove. Cut the chicken into chunks and add them to the glaze; cover, keeping the heat very low.

- Let the chicken poach for 8 to 10 minutes, covered. This ensures that your chicken will be cooked through.

- If you are serving the salad with rice, drizzle the salad with the poaching liquid.

MEDITERRANEAN SEAFOOD SALAD

At lunch or dinner, this salad epitomizes the healthy Mediterranean diet

With this recipe, the more varieties of seafood you use, the better it tastes. Be sure to save the cooking liquids to add to rice or cooked mini pasta shells for added flavor.

You can choose any combination of mollusks and crustaceans. Be sure to serve clams and mussels in their shells. You are not likely, however, to find oysters in a seafood salad; somehow, they just don't quite fit. There is no law, though, saying you can't add a few shucked oysters, raw or poached, to the salad. Be careful, however, when you consume raw shellfish, as bad ones can lead to illness. You don't need to buy jumbo shrimp or diver scallops. Medium shrimp and bay scallops are just fine and far less expensive. *Yield: 4 servings*

Ingredients

¹/₃ cup fresh lemon juice

¹/₃ cup olive oil

1 teaspoon Worcestershire sauce

¹/₄ cup fresh parsley, finely chopped

Salt and pepper to taste

12 littleneck clams

16 mussels

1 cup bay scallops

16 medium shrimp, shelled and deveined

¹/₂ box (8 ounces) small shell pasta, cooked, or 2 cups brown rice

2 cups leafy green lettuce

Garnish: avocados, capers, or fennel leaves

Calories 552, **Fat** (g) 22, **Carbohydrates** (g) 49, **Protein** (g) 38, **Fiber** (g) 2, **Saturated Fat** (g) 3, **Cholesterol** (mg) 168, **Sodium** (mg) 689, **Carb Choices** 3, **ADA Exchange** 3 starch, 4 lean meat, 2 fat

Mediterranean Seafood Salad

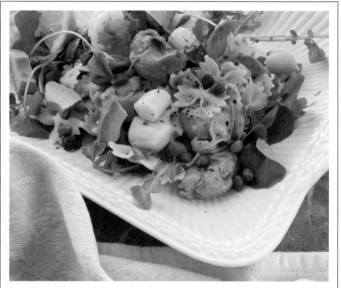

- Mix first five ingredients together to make dressing.

- Scrub closed clams, mussels under cold running water. Discard open shellfish. Place ½ cup water in a pot over high heat. Add shellfish; cover and allow them to steam open. Transfer them to a separate bowl.

- Reduce heat to medium; add scallops, shrimp. Cook 2 minutes, removing when shrimp turns pink.

- Combine cooked seafood. Pour half of dressing over warm seafood. Add rest to cooked pasta or rice. Top greens with pasta or rice, and seafood. Garnish.

Artichoke heart salad: A delicious variation of this recipe is to add a box of frozen baby artichoke hearts. Simply cook them according to package directions. Make one change: acidulate the water. This means that you add 1 table-spoon of lemon juice or vinegar to the cooking liquid to remove any of the bitterness in the artichokes. Marinate the cooked, drained artichokes in citrus dressing and let them "cook" overnight in the refrigerator. Add to salad the next day.

Avocado salad: Another excellent addition to this entrée salad would be avocados. You can slice 2 ripe avocados over the top or arrange slices around the salad. Remember to brush them with fresh lemon or lime juice to prevent them from browning

Use Safe Seafood

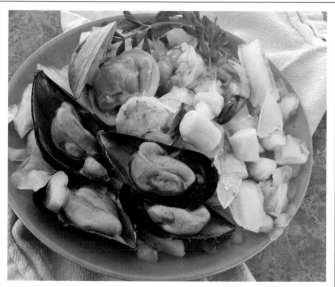

Overcooked Seafood

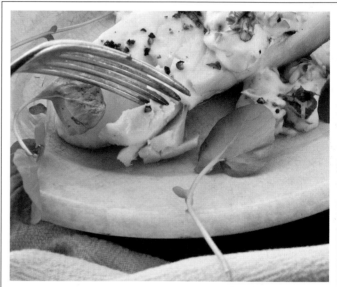

- When cooking with seafood, the first rule is to never use anything that smells even slightly sour or "off."

- Find a really good fish market or a supermarket with a knowledgeable fish department.

- Ask the fishmonger to tap the clams and mussels together to make sure they close up tightly.

- If a clam or mussel makes a dull thud or hollow sound more than once, discard it.

- If you overcook fin fish, it will disintegrate into tiny flakes. This is not attractive and has a mushy texture if poached. Broiled, over-cooked fish will dry out.

- Tuna hardens and salmon loses flavor and moisture when overcooked. Cook until it just begins to flake.

- If you overcook scallops, shrimp, mussels, oysters, or lobster, they will get rubbery.

- Calamari, which is the Italian name for squid, must be cooked only until just barely hot, or cooked a long time, as in 4 hours in a sauce.

GRILLED VEGETABLE SALAD

Whenever you fire up the grill, cook lots of veggies to have on hand for later

Vegetables can be treated with lots of herbs and spices when grilled. They must first be brushed with a little olive oil before going on the grill—that's mandatory.

When working with veggies, use the small varieties of eggplant. Some are actually the size of eggs, while others are about 6 inches long and skinny. Although all eggplant skins are edible, you might not enjoy the large ones. The small varieties have tender skins. Red and green bell peppers need to be peeled if they char. Zucchini and yellow summer squash are just fine—skin and all. Tomatoes are terrific grilled but should have some foil underneath to keep the juices from running into the fire. *Yield: 6 servings*

KNACK DIABETES COOKBOOK

Ingredients

2 tablespoons olive oil

2 cloves garlic, smashed and minced

1 tablespoon dried basil or 3 tablespoons fresh basil

1 tablespoon dried oregano or 3 tablespoons fresh oregano

1 teaspoon hot pepper sauce, or to taste

1/4 cup red wine vinegar

2 sweet red peppers, cut into quarters and cleaned

3 small zucchini, trimmed and cut lengthwise

3 small eggplants, trimmed and cut in half lengthwise

3 tomatoes, cored and cut into thick slices

18 thin asparagus stalks, trimmed

1 large head romaine lettuce, washed, dried, and shredded

18 Italian or Greek olives

12 (4 ounces) small marble-sized balls fresh mozzarella cheese

Calories 176, **Fat** (g) 10, **Carbohydrates** (g) 18, **Protein** (g) 9, **Fiber** (g) 8, **Saturated Fat** (g) 3, **Cholesterol** (mg) 8, **Sodium** (mg) 219, **Carb Choice** 1, **ADA Exchange** 3 vegetable, 2 fat

Grilled Vegetable Salad

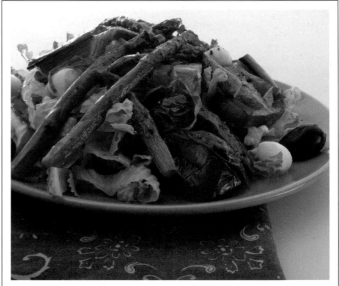

- Fire up the grill or preheat the broiler. Whisk first six ingredients together to make dressing.

- Prepare vegetables, brushing lightly with dressing. Carve tracks into eggplant so dressing can soak in. Place tomato slices on heavy-duty aluminum foil.

- Grill veggies until crisp-tender. Timing depends on grill or kitchen broiler. If peppers are charred, peel them.

- Make a generous bed of greens on a platter; arrange veggies on top. Garnish with olives and fresh mozzarella. Pour any leftover dressing over top.

MAKE IT EASY

The health benefits of asparagus: Asparagus offers plenty of health benefits for people with diabetes. It is high in vitamin K and folate. Its high amounts of folic acid may help prevent some forms of heart disease and strokes. Eating regular amounts of asparagus may also help you lower your cholesterol and fight off high blood pressure.

ZOOM

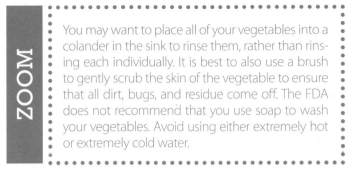

You may want to place all of your vegetables into a colander in the sink to rinse them, rather than rinsing each individually. It is best to also use a brush to gently scrub the skin of the vegetable to ensure that all dirt, bugs, and residue come off. The FDA does not recommend that you use soap to wash your vegetables. Avoid using either extremely hot or extremely cold water.

Washing and Drying Vegetables

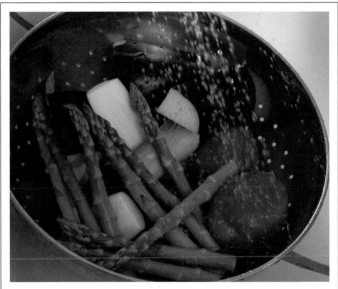

- Wash uncooked vegetables to remove germs and dirt, pesticides, or fertilizer clinging to them.

- Dry the vegetables (air-dry or with paper towels) before grilling them so that the oil and herbs will cling.

- Otherwise, the dressing will simply slide off and puddle into your grill or under your broiler.

- All of the vegetables in this recipe can be placed directly on the grill rack or on a broiler pan in the oven.

Storing Grilled Vegetables

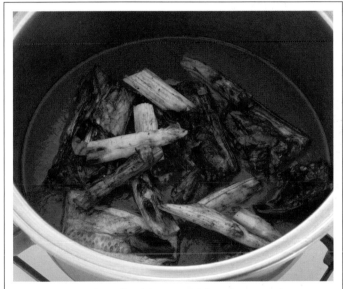

- Grilled vegetables should be used within a day or two. You can keep them in the refrigerator for a couple days, but freezing them will turn them mushy.

- You can actually chop the grilled vegetables and add them to pasta sauce or soup. That will freeze quite well.

- However, the fresh taste of vegetables right off the grill is unbeatable.

TOFU & BROCCOLI SALAD

An Asian-style dressing takes this vegetarian salad from ordinary to extraordinary

The more you cook with tofu, the easier it becomes. And when you add the crunch of nuts and broccoli to the satiny quality of tofu, the better the meal.

Asian dressing is easy to make and adds the finishing touch to a complete dish. However, you can vary the ingredients and come up with something more Italian if you prefer.

Broccoli is one of the so-called power foods, and it is simple to prepare. Tofu is packed with protein, as it comes from soybeans. It is available in firm, extra firm, and satin varieties. For this recipe, try using the satin. For frying and cooking, use the firm or extra firm. *Yield: 6 servings*

Ingredients

2 tablespoons peanut oil

1 tablespoon Asian sesame seed oil

Juice of $1/2$ fresh lemon

2 tablespoons sherry vinegar

1 teaspoon homemade mustard (see recipe, page 208)

1 teaspoon fresh gingerroot

3 tablespoons light soy sauce

$1/2$ cup sweet white onions, finely chopped

1 broccoli crown, divided into florets, microwaved in $1/2$ cup water for 4 minutes on high, then drained

1 pound satin tofu, cubed

$1/4$ cup toasted pine nuts

$1/4$ pound small pasta, cooked (optional)

(Note: This salad can be served warm or chilled.)

Calories 306, **Fat** (g) 22, **Carbohydrates** (g) 17, **Protein** (g) 16, **Fiber** (g) 5, **Saturated Fat** (g) 3, **Cholesterol** (mg) 0, **Sodium** (mg) 359, **Carb Choice** 1, **ADA Exchange** 3 vegetable, 1 medium-fat meat, 3 fat

Tofu & Broccoli Salad

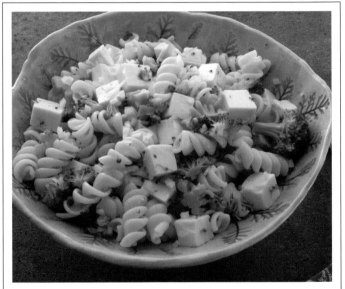

- Whisk first seven ingredients together to make dressing.

- Place all salad ingredients in a large serving bowl and pour on the dressing. Mix well.

- Serve immediately if you want it warm, or chill for later.

92

With napa cabbage and shrimp: Instead of using broccoli, shred napa cabbage for a crunchy alternative. Mix ½ cup light mayonnaise with the Asian dressing for a creamy texture that goes well with cabbage. For added variety, add ½ pound of cooked shrimp to the tofu and cabbage version of this recipe. If you prefer, add ½ pound of chicken or crabmeat. Garnish the salad with ¼ pound of sugar snaps, blanched, rinsed, dried, and cut diagonally.

Italian-style: Then, there's the Italian version of this recipe. You can totally change the flavor of this salad by simply changing the dressing. Use basic red wine vinaigrette or a vinaigrette made with champagne or other white wine. With the broccoli, add some chopped roasted red pepper and ½ cup crumbled Gorgonzola cheese.

Broccoli for Salad or Dinner

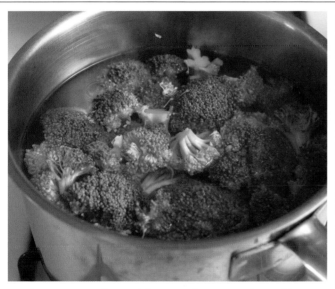

Pasta/Noodles in Salad

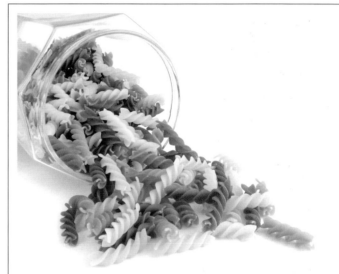

- When preparing broccoli for salad, you generally cook it for a shorter period of time than for a dinner side dish to maintain the crunch.

- Uncooked broccoli can be harsh on the digestive system, producing stomachaches and gas.

- If you are serving older adults or very young children, it's best to cook the broccoli until crisp/tender.

- Or if your dinner table includes elderly people, cook the broccoli for an extra 5 minutes.

- If you are using Asian noodles, you will find that they are much more delicate than regular noodles or pasta.

- Asian noodles are often labeled "glass" or "cellophane" noodles.

- Of course, you can use any noodle or pasta that you like in a salad. However, cook the pasta al dente because it will absorb dressing and get softer as it does so.

- Check out the various kinds of Asian noodles available, and learn to enjoy many different types.

SHRIMP SALAD WITH CASHEWS

You can use other nuts in this recipe, but cashews go especially well with shrimp

This delicious combination will take any home cook a long way. Serve it to a friend for lunch or dinner, or as part of a buffet at a family party whenever you need a lovely dish that's easy to make the day before.

Lime juice is essential in this recipe to counterbalance the sweetness of the cashews. The counterpoint of sweet and tart is what makes cooking interesting. Make this recipe with cold cooked rice or small pasta shells. However, whenever you use a carb such as rice or pasta, make extra sauce and dress it well before serving time, as the noodles or rice will soak up the dressing, and make sure to count the carbs in your meal plan. *Yield: 4 servings*

Ingredients

²/₃ cup low-fat mayonnaise

Juice of 1 fresh lime

1 teaspoon mustard

Salt and freshly ground white or black pepper to taste

¹/₄ cup fresh parsley, finely chopped

1 pound medium shrimp, shelled and deveined

2 stalks celery, finely chopped

¹/₂ cup roasted cashew nuts

4 cups salad greens, such as romaine, iceberg, or baby spinach

Shrimp Salad with Cashews

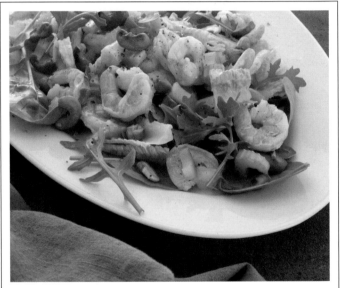

- Mix the mayonnaise, lime juice, mustard, parsley, salt, and pepper together in a bowl.

- Defrost frozen shrimp under cool running water and check for remaining shells. If you are using jumbo shrimp, slice them in half.

- Mix together all of the ingredients except the greens.

- Cover and chill for serving later, or arrange over greens and serve immediately.

Calories 313, **Fat** (g) 17, **Carbohydrates** (g) 15, **Protein** (g) 26, **Fiber** (g) 2, **Saturated Fat** (g) 3, **Cholesterol** (mg) 173, **Sodium** (mg) 345, **Carb Choice** 1, **ADA Exchange** 1 starch, 3 lean meat, 1 fat

MAKE IT EASY

Cooking with cashews: Cashews have a mellow, sweet flavor. They are great chopped and pressed into salmon that's to be grilled or broiled, or you can grind them up and sprinkle them over peaches before you grill them. Cashews also are an excellent counterpoint to shrimp, as in this salad. Do not buy salted cashews. The last thing anyone, much less a person with diabetes, needs to consume is extraneous salt. Just get raw or roasted cashews and start adding them to other salads, meat, and vegetable dishes. Try adding cashews to any chicken dish, such as chicken salad. Baked chicken, even chicken potpie, will benefit greatly from the addition of a cup of cashews. They add crunch and interest to what could be an otherwise bland dish.

Choosing Shrimp for Salad

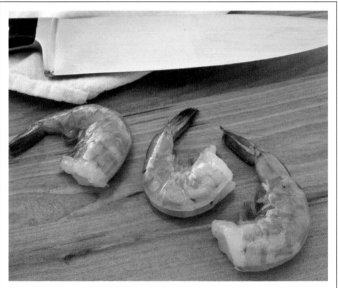

- Freshly netted Gulf shrimp is a luxury unless you live right along the Gulf of Mexico and know the friendly owner of a shrimp boat.

- Any extra-large to jumbo shrimp has to be cut into bite-size pieces. You don't want your guests to have to use a knife to cut up their salad.

- Although shrimp has a bad reputation because it is high in dietary cholesterol, it is very low in saturated fat, so, it's a great source of lean protein. Just don't eat it every day.

Peeling and Cleaning Shrimp

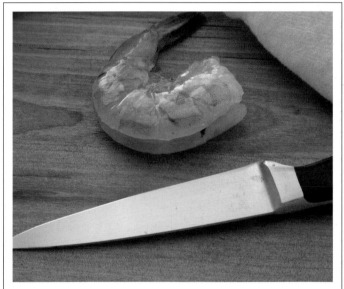

- Fresh or defrosted shrimp is easy to peel; in fact, you can use a shrimp-peeling gadget, which makes it faster.

- First, pull off the legs and remove the shell.

- Then, with a very sharp knife, make a shallow cut along the back and remove any black intestines.

- Rinse the shrimp thoroughly to remove all the grit. Poach the shrimp (in wine or beer) until it turns pink. Drain, chill, and use in your salad.

GRILLED ASPARAGUS

You can make the same grilled asparagus that is served in many upscale restaurants

Antioxidants are incredibly important to your health because they kill cancer-causing free radicals. All green vegetables, including asparagus, have antioxidants.

Asparagus can be grilled indoors or out. If you are grilling it outside on a charcoal or gas grill, be sure to skewer the spears together with metal or wooden skewers. If you use wooden skewers, soak them in water for an hour, or the heat of the grill will burn them. Asparagus is especially nice with either melted butter and lemon vinaigrette or Hollandaise sauce. Or eat them plain with a bit of low-fat mayo. Thick asparagus is tender and juicy but needs its ends peeled. Thin asparagus does not need peeling. *Yield: 4 servings*

Ingredients

16–24 fresh asparagus spears

1 cup of your favorite vinaigrette

Grilled Asparagus

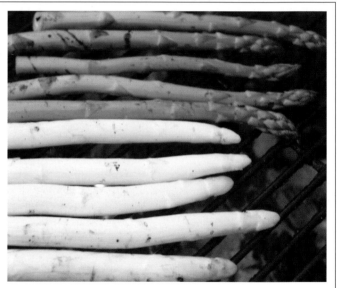

- Break off and discard the tough ends of the asparagus. Wash and dry on paper towels.

- Place the asparagus in a flat pan and add the vinaigrette.

- Marinate the asparagus for 30 minutes to 2 hours.

- Preheat grill to 350°F. Grill quickly, until just beginning to brown. Serve hot, at room temperature, or cold.

Calories 64, **Fat** (g) 4, **Carbohydrates** (g) 7, **Protein** (g) 2, **Fiber** (g) 2, **Saturated Fat** (g) 0, **Cholesterol** (mg) 4, **Sodium** (mg) 822, **ADA Exchange** 1 vegetable, 1 fat

Use asparagus in soups, salads, or as a side green. Or wrap it in light whole-wheat bread with a cheese spread, cut in small pieces, and bake for appetizers. Cook it quickly in the microwave. Cut it in lengths that fit your bowl. Add 2 tablespoons water, 1 tablespoon low-fat margarine, and some lemon juice. Cover with paper. Depending on the level of doneness you like, microwave 2 to 5 minutes on high.

Marinate your veggies: Any citrus vinaigrette or white wine vinaigrette will work as a marinade. If you marinate in mustardy BBQ sauce, keep it farther from the flame when cooking or it will burn. String 18 to 24 (depending on size) mushrooms on 4 separate skewers and coat with marinade; serve them in addition to the asparagus in a salad over cooked rice or pasta as a side dish.

Trimming Asparagus Ends

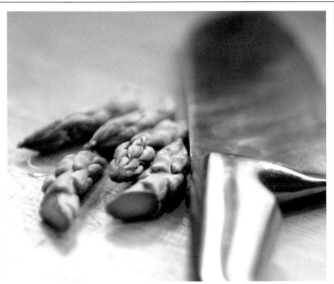

Green or White Asparagus?

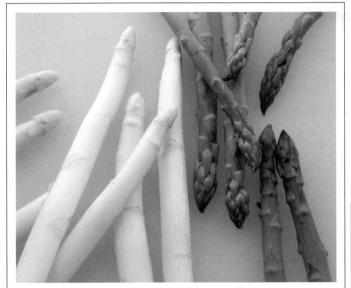

- Remove the tough, woody ends from stalks of asparagus.

- Using a potato peeler, simply start peeling where the asparagus gets thick but is still green.

- Peel thick stalks if nubby or 1 inch in diameter at the widest. Only peel the green part; discard the white or purple ends.

- Break off the end of one stalk, then line it up the rest. Using it as a guide, cut the rest of the stems with a knife.

- Although white asparagus is considered a gourmet delicacy, try to get the greenest produce in the market.

- White asparagus is white because it is light-deprived; no sun touches it. Therefore, the vegetable does not make chlorophyll.

- Chlorophyll is the product of photosynthesis; plants turn light into chlorophyll, which gives them their green color.

- There are a lot more vitamins and minerals in green asparagus than in the white, which is grown under a tent or pot.

GREEN VEGETABLES

BROCCOLI WITH GARLIC SAUCE

Broccoli is a "power" food because it's packed with nutrients

From florets to stems, broccoli is a superfood. Use the florets for your green vegetable sides, salads, and snacks. Use the stems for soup.

Broccoli is a member of the crucifer family of vegetables, which also include brussels sprouts, broccolini, broccoli rabe, and various forms of cabbage. All of these vegetables are full of antioxidants, which fight cancer by literally killing off the free radicals we get from other sources.

Garlic is a very healthful aromatic herb and goes very well with broccoli. Garlic in a little oil or low-fat margarine, or mixed with vinaigrette, enhances the flavors of vegetables whether they are cooked or raw. It's strongest when minced, mildest when whole or cut into large slices. *Yield: 4 servings*

Ingredients

2 tablespoons lemon juice

2 tablespoons olive oil

2 cloves garlic, smashed and slivered

Salt and pepper to taste

1 pound broccoli, separated into small florets, stems set aside

Broccoli with Garlic Sauce

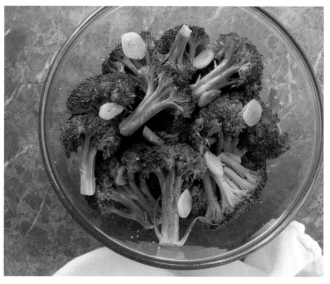

- Place the first 4 ingredients in a glass bowl and mix.

- Rinse the broccoli but do not dry it. Swish it around in the lemon-oil-garlic mixture.

- Cover with freezer paper or paper towels.

- Microwave 2 minutes. Turn the broccoli and microwave another 2 to 4 minutes, depending on desired level of tenderness.

Calories 91, **Fat** (g) 7, **Carbohydrates** (g) 5, **Protein** (g) 2, **Fiber** (g) 0, **Saturated Fat** (g) 3, **Cholesterol** (mg) 0, **Sodium** (mg) 20, **ADA Exchange** 1 vegetable, 1 fat

Broccoli and citrus: This recipe is very quick and delicious, as well as being nutritious. Add 1 tablespoon of fresh lime juice to garlic sauce, omitting the lemon juice. One teaspoon of lemon zest adds flavor. The reconstituted stuff does not work as well. If some members of your family like the broccoli to be more crisp, simply microwave some of the broccoli for 2 minutes and the rest of the broccoli for 4 minutes.

Boiling broccoli: A second method of cooking is to drop the broccoli into boiling, lightly salted water. Cook for 5 minutes, then remove from the cooking water. Shock by plunging it into ice water; drain. Make your sauce in a large sauté pan over medium heat. Add the broccoli to the sauce on top of the stove.

Preparing Broccoli Stems for Soup

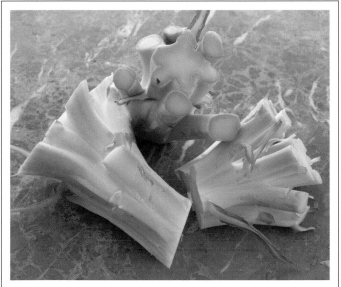

- Wash the stems. Cut ⅛ inch off the very bottom of each stem.

- Cut the broccoli stems crossways, into ¼-inch "coins."

- Cook the coins in boiling salted water or light chicken broth, enough to cover.

- Sauté 1 onion and 2 cloves garlic until soft. Add to the soup ½ teaspoon each thyme and oregano for flavor. Cool the soup, and then blend in batches in a food processor or blender.

Another Broccoli-Like Vegetable

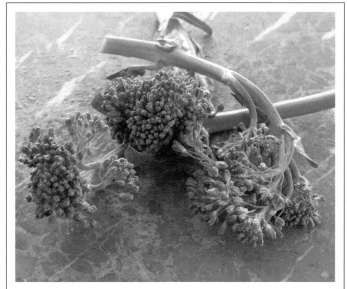

- Broccolini is not, as most people think, very young broccoli. It is a hybrid, a cross between broccoli and a Chinese cabbage called kai lan.

- It was developed in Japan and has become very popular worldwide because of its pleasant flavor and high nutritional content.

- You can cook broccolini exactly the way you would cook broccoli. Because it's smaller, it takes less time.

- Broccollini is tender and delicious, and high in vitamin A, calcium, and iron.

GREEN VEGETABLES

99

BROCCOLI RABE WITH PASTA
Fans of this slightly bitter vegetable claim it is positively addictive

Broccoli rabe, or rapini, is also know as "rape" and is beloved by the Italians, Spanish, and Portuguese. It's blanched and then sautéed in oil, butter, or low-fat margarine.

Broccoli rabe looks a lot like broccoli; however, you do eat the stems and leaves. It has a slightly bitter or pungent flavor, which is lessened by blanching. It's very popular in Italian restaurants as a side dish or as a main course with sweet or

hot sausage. It's also popular on pizza, where it is precooked by blanching, mixed with two or three kinds of cheese, and baked on the crust.

This recipe can make an entire meal because it has protein from the cheese, carbs from the pasta, and vegetables. *Yield: 6 servings*

Ingredients

1 pound broccoli rabe, washed and chopped into 1-inch pieces

1 pound low-fat ricotta cheese

$^{1}/_{2}$ cup Parmesan cheese. finely grated

1 egg, slightly beaten

$^{1}/_{4}$ teaspoon nutmeg

Juice of $^{1}/_{2}$ lemon

Freshly ground black pepper to taste

$^{1}/_{2}$ pound whole-wheat pasta

$^{1}/_{4}$ cup extra-virgin olive oil

1 teaspoon dried oregano

Calories 380, **Fat** (g) 18, **Carbohydrates** (g) 35, **Protein** (g) 21, **Fiber** (g) 5, **Saturated Fat** (g) 7, **Cholesterol** (mg) 31, **Sodium** (mg) 275, **Carb Choices** 2, **ADA Exchange** 2 starch, 1 vegetable, 1 medium-fat protein, 2 fat

Broccoli Rabe with Pasta

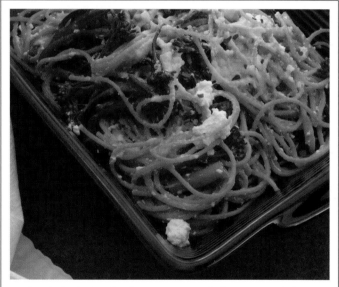

- Blanch the broccoli rabe 3 minutes in boiling water; place in colander to drain.

- Mix the ricotta, Parmesan, egg, nutmeg, and pepper together in a bowl. Add lemon juice.

- Cook the pasta and drain; place in a large, ovenproof serving bowl. Toss the olive oil and oregano with the pasta.

- Add the broccoli rabe and the cheese mixture. Mix well and bake for 20 minutes at 325°F.

Always blanch broccoli rabe: Unless your taste buds are very well conditioned, always blanch broccoli rabe for a couple minutes in boiling water to remove the bitterness. And remember, you can and should eat the leaves and stems, too. After blanching, you can cut it into 1- to 2-inch segments for sautéing as a side, mixing with other ingredients, or spreading on a white pizza. If sautéing, do so with garlic and a drop of olive oil, then sprinkle it with lemon juice. You can also use shallots instead of, or in addition to, garlic.

Blanching Vegetables

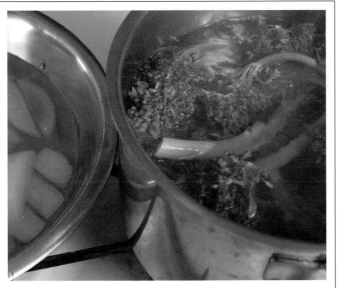

- You can blanch any green vegetable to keep it crisp/tender; then, shock it to keep it a bright green.

- Bring a large pot of water to a rolling boil. You can add a little salt, but it's not necessary.

- Immerse the vegetables in the boiling water. Return to a boil and cook for 1 to 5 minutes, depending on the kind of vegetable and the level on doneness you want.

- Drain.

Shocking Vegetables

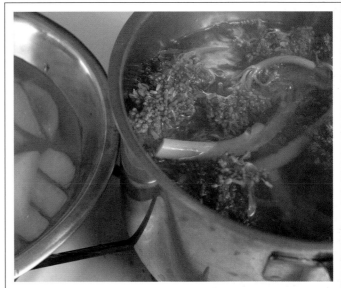

- After blanching, shock your vegetables to stop the cooking and brighten the green. Drain, then plunge them into a bowl of ice water to shock them.

- Don't blanch and shock spinach; it will turn limp and watery.

- Blanch and shock green beans, asparagus, broccoli rabe, broccoli, broccolini, and artichokes (prior to baking).

- Blanching and shocking prior to sautéing vegetables also tenderizes them.

GREEN VEGETABLES

101

SAUCY GREEN BEANS

These green beans soar to new heights with a little freshly made tomato sauce

Green beans are great for mixing with other goodies. They go well with nuts, mushrooms, garlic, shallots, and, in the case of this recipe, fresh cherry tomatoes made into a quick sauce.

Always blanch and shock green beans (see techniques on page 101). They will stay crisp/tender and very green. Then, add them to a sauce, sauté them, or even use fresh green beans for cream of mushroom soup and onion casserole (a dish that should be enjoyed in moderation). Freshly blanched and shocked green beans give a finer flavor to this dish. Since fresh green beans are available year-round, the only reason to use frozen ones is convenience. *Yield: 6 servings*

Ingredients

1 pound fresh cherry tomatoes, rinsed and stemmed

2 tablespoons olive oil

2 cloves garlic, smashed, peeled, and sliced

2 shallots, peeled and sliced

1 pound green string beans, trimmed

1 teaspoon dried rosemary or 1 tablespoon fresh rosemary

1 teaspoon dried oregano or 1 tablespoon fresh oregano

Salt and freshly ground black pepper to taste

Garnish: 2 tablespoons freshly grated Parmesan cheese

Calories 94, **Fat** (g) 5, **Carbohydrates** (g) 11, **Protein** (g) 3, **Fiber** (g) 4, **Saturated Fat** (g) 1, **Cholesterol** (mg) 2, **Sodium** (mg) 30, **ADA Exchange** 2 vegetable, 1 fat

Saucy Green Beans

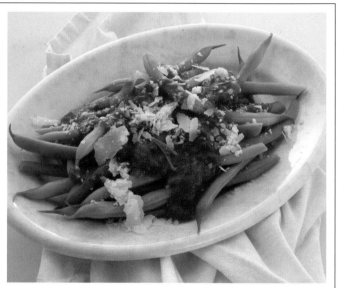

- Place half of the tomatoes in a blender and puree; add the other half and puree until very fine. Set aside.

- Heat olive oil over medium heat in a large sauté pan; add garlic and shallots. Sauté, stirring to cook evenly. Add the tomatoes to the pan and cover;

reduce heat to low.

- Blanch and shock the beans; drain.

- Add the beans, herbs, salt, and pepper to the pot of tomato sauce. Cover and cook 5 minutes. Sprinkle with cheese and serve.

Storing your beans: Green beans store well in the refrigerator and can also be frozen for future use. If freezing, wash them first and then dry thoroughly. Prepare a cookie sheet with nonstick spray. Place the beans on the cookie sheet, making sure they are not touching, and put them in the freezer for about 45 minutes. Quickly place handfuls of beans in storage bags, seal tightly, and put right back into the freezer. Of course, there is nothing wrong with commercially frozen green beans, but they are never as crisp as the ones you freeze yourself. Plus, if you have a garden full of green beans, you have the satisfaction of eating food you've grown, tended, and lovingly prepared.

Why Your Sauce Turns Pink

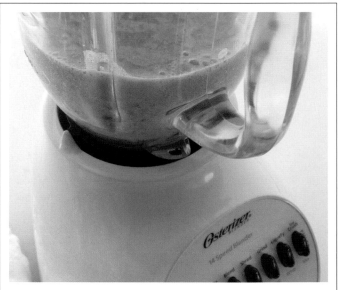

- When you puree tomatoes in a blender, they turn pink. This is because the air and water dilute the tomatoes.

- Don't worry; you won't end up with a pink tomato sauce.

- Just let it cook for a while, and it will change back to a true red. This foolproof technique can also be used for a soup base.

- Tomatoes vary in juiciness. Mix the base with 1 tablespoon tomato paste to thicken, or with 1 cup chicken or beef broth if too thick.

Dried vs. Fresh Herbs

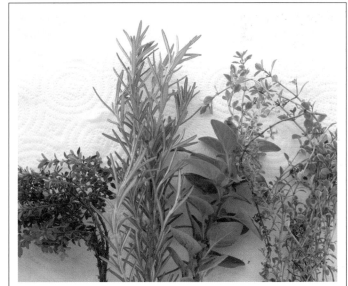

- Fresh herbs are full of moisture. Flavors are concentrated in dried herbs.

- That's why you use two or three times the amount of fresh herbs compared to dried herbs.

- Use your dried herbs as soon as possible. They lose their power and aroma when stored for months on end.

- This is not as true of spices, such as nutmeg, cloves, and cinnamon. They hold their flavors longer.

COLLARD GREENS IN BROTH

A staple of Southern cooking, collards are an excellent source of fiber

Collard greens are a standard of Southern cooking. They are easy to grow and extremely healthful. Collards are ideal for people with diabetes because they are not only low in carb, but also a great source of fiber, calcium, and iron.

Collards, like kale, have a heavy stem and tend to be sandy. Lots of cooks buy the frozen greens because they don't require so much prep work. Collards can be garnished with crumbled bacon (turkey bacon is recommended), bits of smoked ham, and herbs.

Collard greens need a fair amount of cooking. You can cook them in any kind of broth, though ham hock broth is traditional. Collards can be substituted for kale or turnip greens in soups and stews. They go especially well with ham or pork chops. *Yield: 6 servings*

Ingredients

1 large bunch of collard greens, cleaned and torn into small pieces and reserved

¼ cup olive oil

2 cloves garlic, smashed, peeled, and sliced

2 medium onions, peeled and chopped

¼ pound smoked turkey (used in analysis) or turkey bacon, chopped into small pieces

2 cups broth (chicken or vegetable)

1 tablespoon cider vinegar

Salt and pepper to taste

Calories 160, **Fat** (g) 13, **Carbohydrates** (g) 6, **Protein** (g) 6, **Fiber** (g) 1, **Saturated Fat** (g) 2, **Cholesterol** (mg) 14, **Sodium** (mg) 453, **ADA Exchange** 1 vegetable, 3 fat

Collard Greens in Broth

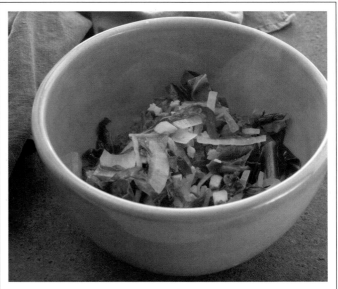

- In a large soup pot, heat the oil over medium setting. Add garlic, onions, and smoked turkey or turkey bacon; sauté for five minutes.

- Add the reserved greens; stir to coat well. Add the broth, vinegar, salt, and pepper.

- Cover and simmer on low for 45 minutes or until very tender.

Easy cleaning: The best way to get the sand, dirt, and grit out of collards is to remove the heavy stems and break up the greens. Then, fill a sink with cold water, add the greens, swoosh them around, and put them in a colander. You can spin them dry or leave them wet, depending on whether you are planning to braise or poach them.

Southern recipes call for sautéing collard greens in bacon fat and then cooking them in ham hock broth. That's a lot of extra calories and fat that people with diabetes must avoid. Instead, sauté the collard greens with cooked turkey bacon if you are craving a down-home experience.

Greens Runneth Over? That's OK!

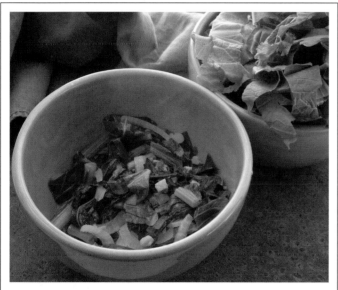

- It may look as though you have too many greens for this recipe. You don't. All greens (spinach, kale, collards, etc.) cook down, and down, and down.

- The trick is to start by cooking half of them, stirring until they reduce in size.

- Keep adding greens a handful at a time, until you've mixed them all in with the broth.

- Cover and simmer until tender.

Poaching vs. Braising

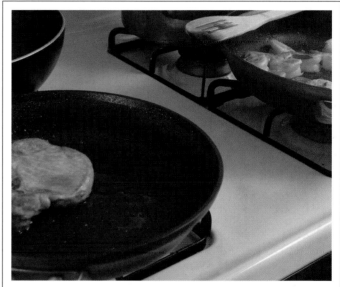

- Poaching works well for many things, among them eggs, salmon, and asparagus.

- You poach by gently lowering food into hot liquid, and then cooking it very, very slowly.

- Braising is a bit different. You start by sautéing meat, fish, or poultry, then you add liquid.

- At this point, you reduce the heat and cover the pot or pan. The food then cooks for a long time, until it is tender. Perfect for collard greens!

GREEN VEGETABLES

ZUCCHINI-TOMATO CASSEROLE

Here's what to do with all that zucchini from the summer garden

Zucchini abounds in summer gardens, and those who grow it always seem to have too much. Friends with gardens will put it in your mailbox, on the seat of your car, on your back doorstep.

However, it's wonderful in soup and bread and as a simple veggie side dish. This recipe has everything you need for a meal.

There are many ways to add extra nutrition to this recipe. When you are layering the sausage and zucchini, you can add a layer of white beans or chickpeas. Layering with two or three different cheeses is another way to make this casserole a bit richer and more delicious. *Yield: 6 servings*

Ingredients

2 tablespoons olive oil

1 teaspoon garlic powder

Salt and pepper to taste

1 tablespoon dried basil or 3 tablespoons fresh basil, shredded

2 teaspoons dried oregano or 4 teaspoons fresh oregano

1 tablespoon dried rosemary or 2 tablespoons fresh rosemary

1 tablespoons olive oil

2 medium zucchini, trimmed and thinly sliced

1 large onion, peeled and thinly sliced

4 ripe tomatoes, thinly sliced, or 1 cup tomato sauce

1 13-ounce can white or pink beans, rinsed and drained

1 cup seasoned bread crumbs

¹/₂ cup grated Parmesan cheese

Calories 304, **Fat** (g) 12, **Carbohydrates** (g) 34, **Protein** (g) 16, **Fiber** (g) 5, **Saturated Fat** (g) 7, **Cholesterol** (mg) 63, **Sodium** (mg) 1641, **Carb Choices** 2, **ADA Exchange** 2 starch, 1 vegetable, 1½ medium-fat meat, 1 fat

Zucchini-Tomato Casserole

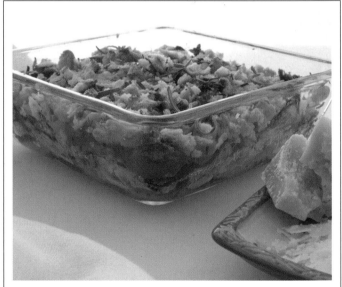

- Preheat oven to 350°F. Mix 2 tablespoons oil, garlic powder, salt, pepper, and herbs together.

- Prepare a 2-quart casserole with nonstick spray. Layer half of the zucchini, onion, and tomato. Spread with

beans. Top with the rest of the veggies. Drizzle with the oil and herb mixture. Sprinkle with bread crumbs and Parmesan.

- Bake at 350°F for 25 minues or until the casserole sizzles and the top is golden.

• • • • RECIPE VARIATION • • • •

Fun variations: This casserole provides great flexibility. The more goodies you add, the more people it will feed. You can use yellow summer squash instead of green zucchini. It looks very pretty and has a buttery flavor. Parmesan cheese is essential, but you can layer slices of mozzarella, Muenster, or other low-fat cheese.

Tomatoes or sauce? Use fresh tomatoes or tomato sauce, your own or bottled. Or use a can of crushed tomatoes—just be sure to sprinkle extra fresh herbs over them. If you use canned tomatoes, use extra seasoned bread crumbs to soak up some of the moisture from the tomatoes. Commercial pasta sauces can be heavily seasoned; if you use a jar, taste it before you add any additional seasonings.

How to Layer a Casserole

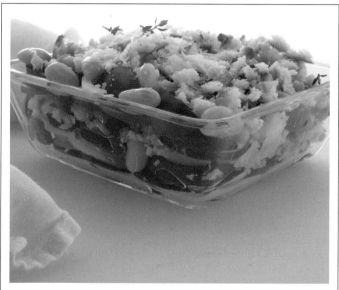

- Because the ingredients range from moist to wet, try to layer in plenty of bread crumbs and things that go well together.

- Add beans between the layer of tomatoes and the layer of zucchini.

- The cheese can go over the tomatoes or between layers.

Make Your Own Breadcrumbs

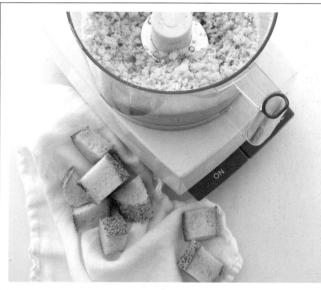

- Dry bread crumbs are a cinch to make. Simply cut some stale French or Italian bread into chunks.

- Put the bread in a food processor or blender. Blend more for fine crumbs or less for coarse crumbs.

- You can add dried herbs, Parmesan cheese, salt, and pepper to the crumbs.

- Store them in an airtight container in the refrigerator.

GREEN VEGETABLES

YELLOW SNAP BEANS

Yellow string beans, snap beans, and wax beans are one and the same

Yellow string beans have a slightly sweet taste. You can cook them in all the same ways that you cook green string beans. They add a bright spot of color to a dinner plate and are as good as green beans in bean salads. Yellow snap beans make an attractive presentation when paired with green herbs and/or tomatoes.

The garnishes for this recipe are fresh summer herbs and toasted walnuts. You can use pecans or almonds; however, buttery walnuts are wonderful.

You might also enjoy mixing yellow and green beans for an even more colorful side dish. This go-with-everything vegetable is a great side with any meat or poultry. *Yield: 4 servings*

Ingredients

1 teaspoon low-fat margarine

$1/3$ cup walnut pieces

1 pound yellow wax beans, trimmed

$1/2$ cup water

1 tablespoon olive oil

6 fresh basil leaves, shredded

2 sprigs fresh rosemary, chopped

Salt and freshly ground pepper to taste

Juice of $1/2$ fresh lemon

Calories 70, **Fat** (g) 4, **Carbohydrates** (g) 9, **Protein** (g) 2, **Fiber** (g) 3, **Saturated Fat** (g) 1, **Cholesterol** (mg) 0, **Sodium** (mg) 11, **ADA Exchange** 2 vegetable, 1 fat

Yellow Snap Beans

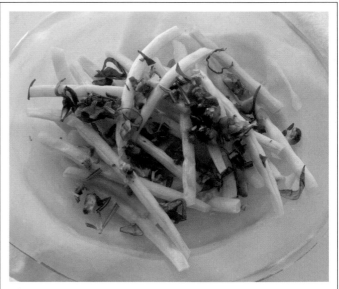

- Heat the low-fat margarine in a nonstick pan. Add walnuts and sauté for 5 minutes, shaking pan, until crisp but not burned.

- In a saucepan, steam beans in the water, covered, for 6 to 10 minutes.

- Drain beans and place in a serving bowl. Toss in olive oil and add herbs.

- Season with salt and pepper; sprinkle with lemon juice. Toss in sautéed walnuts.

Strictly vegetarian: You can make your vegetarian relatives and friends a delicious main course with yellow beans. The formula is simple. Steam the beans lightly and put them in an ovenproof serving bowl that you've prepared with nonstick spray. Add 1 can of black beans, rinsed and drained. (You can also use white beans, pinto beans, or red kidney beans.) Then mix in 6 ounces of salsa and ½ pound of any good sharp white or yellow cheddar cheese or low-fat cheese. Bake for 15 minutes. While still hot, sprinkle with fresh chopped cilantro or Italian flat-leaf parsley. On the side, have plenty of fresh chopped onions. Serve the bean casserole with corn bread or thinly sliced whole-grain bread.

Cutting Your Beans

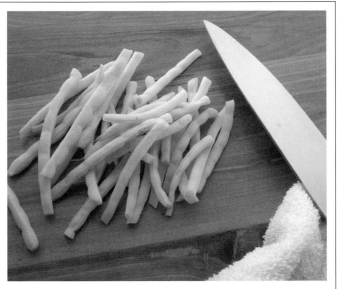

- It is important to trim the stems from the beans. Wait until after the beans are cooked to cut off the pointy ends.

- If you cut the beans into bite-size pieces, more moisture will be depleted than if you leave them whole.

- To trim the stems, line up the beans in batches with all ends in a row. Cut the stems off all in one swipe of the knife.

Microwaving Your Vegetables

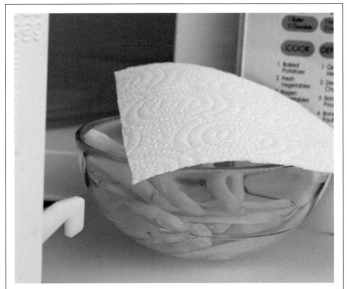

- Boiling, steaming, or microwaving your vegetables is the most healthful way to cook veggies.

- They will actually steam in the microwave. It takes less time, and you have less to clean up.

- Wash the vegetables, then put them in a glass or ceramic bowl with a little water.

- Cover with a paper towel or freezer paper. Microwave on high for 60 seconds; check for doneness and cook longer if necessary.

YELLOW VEGETABLES

BABY BLUE NOSE TURNIPS

Sweeter than most turnips, these are mashed and can be combined with other root veggies

Baby blue nose turnips are vastly different from the big yellow and orange turnips that are available in markets between November and February.

These turnips are approximately 2 to 2½ inches in diameter and are easy to peel. More prevalent in Europe, they are now showing up in American supermarkets, whereas they were only available in specialty stores a few years ago. Many really great recipes from yesteryear call for these turnips to be added to soups and/or stews. This recipe calls for the turnips to be mashed. They are also wonderful mixed with other root vegetables and tubers, such as potatoes, carrots, and parsnips. *Yield: 4 servings*

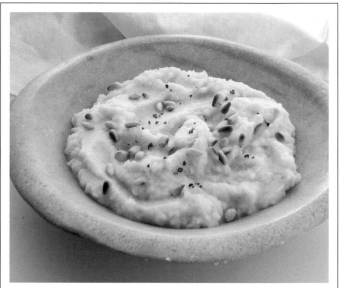

Baby Blue Nose Turnips

Ingredients

1 pound baby blue nose turnips, peeled and sliced

1 carrot, peeled and cut into slices

1 baking potato, peeled and cut into chunks

1 tablespoon low-fat margarine

¹/₂ cup low-fat milk

¹/₂ teaspoon nutmeg

Onion powder to taste

Freshly ground black pepper to taste

¹/₂ cup pine nuts, toasted

- Place the turnips, carrot, and potato in a saucepan with ½ cup of water. Cook over medium-high heat until tender, or microwave on high for 4 minutes.

- Mash the cooked vegetables by hand or with an electric mixer.

- Beat in the margarine, milk, and spices.

- Place the turnip mixture in a nonstick, ovenproof ceramic or glass dish, and sprinkle with toasted pine nuts. Keep warm until ready to serve.

Calories 157, **Fat** (g) 6, **Carbohydrates** (g) 23, **Protein** (g) 4, **Fiber** (g) 4, **Saturated Fat** (g) 1, **Cholesterol** (mg) 1, **Sodium** (mg) 77, **Carb Choices** 1½, **ADA Exchange** 1½ starch, 1 fat

Winter vegetables: Winter veggies are items that keep over the winter. They ripen and can be picked in late September or early October. Native Americans made "root cellars," pits dug into the ground, covered with branches and animal hides to keep hungry scavengers out. Winter vegetables include turnips, carrots, beets, parsnips, potatoes, pumpkins, winter squash, onions, garlic, and a few greens, including cabbage, kale, turnip greens, collards, brussels sprouts, leeks, and broccoli. The vitamins and minerals derived from winter vegetables help us to get through the winter without getting scurvy from the lack of vitamin C.

How to Pick a Blue Nose Turnip

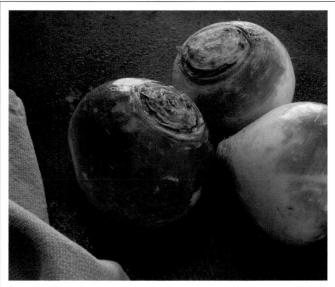

- Look for a turnip with a snowy white body and fresh mauve tip.

- Make sure the stem ends are stiff and very green.

- Squeeze the turnips to make sure they aren't wizened (old and dry).

- Store turnips in your refrigerator vegetable drawer for up to three months.

How to Peel a Turnip

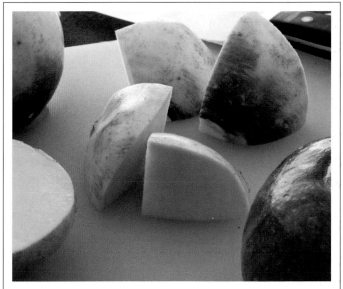

- Using a very sharp knife, remove the stem and root ends of the turnip.

- Cut the turnip crosswise in ⅓-inch rounds.

- Peel off the skin.

- Place in cold salted water until ready to cook.

YUKON GOLD POTATO STRIPS

Baked, not fried, these golden potatoes are appealing to the eye and crisp to the taste

Because they are baked and not fried, these potatoes are fat free, and no fat is added to the dish. These golden-fleshed potatoes can be used any way you would use white potatoes, but they stand up especially well to baking and oven-frying.

Although yellow-gold–fleshed potatoes are common in Europe, they are recent arrivals to North America. Yukon

Golds are a cross between North American white potatoes and wild South American yellow potatoes. They are slightly lower in starch than Idaho, New England, or other russet potatoes. They have a buttery flavor, so they require less butter to taste good. This recipe is good for a dinner side or a game-day party. *Yield: 6 servings*

Ingredients

3 Yukon Gold potatoes, peeled and cut into thin strips

3 egg whites, beaten until stiff

$1/2$ teaspoon garlic powder

$1/2$ teaspoon salt, or to taste

$1/2$ teaspoon freshly ground pepper (white pepper if you have it)

$1/2$ cup cornmeal

Yukon Gold Potato Strips

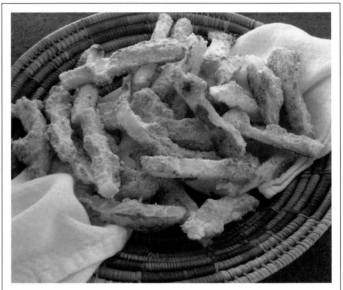

- Preheat oven to 450°F. Cover a baking sheet with aluminum foil; coat the foil with nonstick spray.

- Parboil the potatoes until crisp-tender, about 10 minutes; drain and then dry on paper towels.

- Mix the beaten eggs with garlic powder, salt, pepper, and cornmeal.

- Coat potatoes with the egg mixture and place on baking sheet. Bake for about 8 minutes per side or until crisp on the outside and tender inside.

Calories 180, **Fat** (g) 0, **Carbohydrates** (g) 38, **Protein** (g) 6, **Fiber** (g) 5, **Saturated Fat** (g) 0, **Cholesterol** (mg) 0, **Sodium** (mg) 233, **Carb Choices** 2½, **ADA Exchange** 2½ starch

Scalloping Yukon Gold potatoes: This variation adds a few more calories. Use 1 potato per serving. Spread peeled and sliced potatoes on the bottom of an dish prepared with nonstick spray. Layer with 2 sliced onions, ½ cup bread crumbs, and ½ cup Parmesan cheese. Add ½ cup low-fat milk, and dot with margarine. Bake 1½ hours; serve. Or, add ½ pound cooked turkey sausage, cooked turkey bacon, or low-fat ham in layers between layers of potatoes.

More veggies: To fortify this dish with veggies, add 1 cup of green peas, spinach, or small broccoli florets that have been blanched to the layers of potato and onion. Sprinkle ½ cup grated cheddar cheese over vegetable layer. Use thinly sliced beefsteak or plum tomatoes between the layers of potato, and sprinkle with oregano.

Peeling Yukon Gold Potatoes

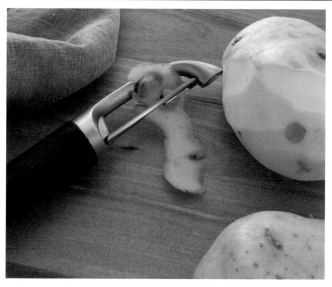

- Run your peeler from end to end when you peel these potatoes, which are more oval and flatter than Idaho potatoes.

- Peeling with a knife wastes a lot of potato.

- The only way to peel a potato with a knife is to cut the strips first, and then carefully slice off the skin.

- The peeler should be really sharp; throw it away when it gets dull.

Slicing: Knife or Mandolin?

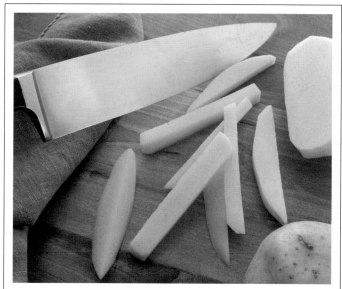

- If you are making potato chips, use a mandolin set at ¹⁄₁₆ inch.

- If you are slicing for scalloped potatoes, use a mandolin set to cut potatoes ⅛-inch thick.

- Some mandolins have handles; those are the ones to get. Otherwise, it's too easy to slice your fingers.

- Use a very sharp knife for making potato strips, and try to cut strips evenly so that they all cook at the same time.

YELLOW VEGETABLES

ACORN SQUASH WITH APPLES

A bit of brown sugar brings out the natural sweetness of acorn squash when roasted

When you roast acorn squash, you have the option of making it sweet or savory, or both at the same time. The savory comes from adding herbs such as sage, rosemary, and thyme. The sweetness is in the squash. A bit of reduced-sugar or sugar-free brown sugar (try Splenda) and low-fat margarine is an excellent seasoning for winter squash.

There are many winter squashes, from butternut to pumpkin, to turban shapes with stripes, confetti, and other interesting markings. They all taste similar, but some are sweeter. Buttercup squash is one of the sweetest. Use a sharp knife to cut any squash. A razor-sharp knife is safer to use than a dull one, which can slip during cutting. *Yield: 4 servings*

Ingredients

2 acorn squash, 1 pound each, cut in half, seeds removed

4 tart apples, such as Granny Smith, peeled and coarsely chopped

$1/4$ teaspoon ground cinnamon

2 tablespoons brown Splenda

2 tablespoons low-fat margarine

Acorn Squash with Apples

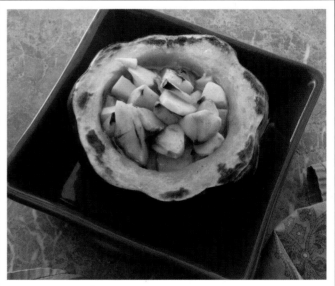

- Par-cook squash either by roasting it in the oven (350°F for 30 minutes) or in the microwave, wrapped in paper, 8 to 10 minutes on high.

- In a saucepan, combine apples, cinnamon, Splenda, and low-fat margarine with 2 tablespoons water.

- Preheat the oven to 350°F. Place squash halves in a baking pan. Add the apple filling to the hollowed-out halves.

- Bake for 35 minutes or until both the squash and apples are soft and steaming hot.

Calories 221, **Fat** (g) 1, **Carbohydrates** (g) 51, **Protein** (g) 2, **Fiber** (g) 7, **Saturated Fat** (g) 0, **Cholesterol** (mg) 0, **Sodium** (mg) 50, **Carb Choices** 3½, **ADA Exchange** 2 starch, 1½ fruit

Once the acorn squash is cut in half, scrape out all of the seeds. Partially bake it at 350°F or microwave for 4 minutes on high to soften it. You can then stuff the squash with any number of delicious fillings. Turkey stuffing made with corn bread is very good. Mix in some cooked sage sausages and apples. Or try making your own multigrain-bread stuffing with lots of herbs, onions, and garlic.

Winter squash comes in bright orange, green, beige, and blended colors. With this recipe for acorn squash, it doesn't really matter whether you get the orange ones or the dark green ones. You do want to get good-size squash because you will be cutting them in half, with one half per person per serving. If all you can get are tiny vegetables, count on a whole one for each serving.

Cutting Squash

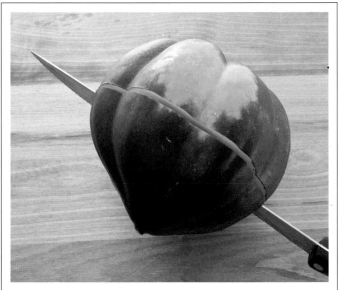

- Cutting up squash can be tiresome and frustrating.

- To eliminate stress, use two knives: a very sharp one to make the initial cut and a serrated knife to saw your way through.

- Wearing a rubber glove to hold the squash steady is also very useful.

- Remember, the sharper the knife, the better.

Roasting Your Seeds

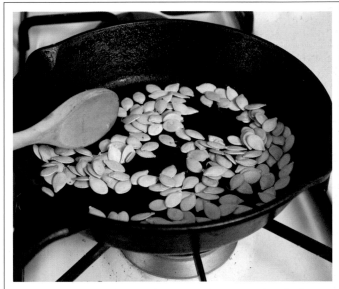

- Squash and pumpkin seeds are very much the same.

- Begin by cleaning the squash or pumpkin seeds under running water to remove strings.

- Dry them thoroughly. Place on a baking sheet that you've covered with aluminum foil and prepared with nonstick spray.

- Toss the seeds in melted low-fat margarine with some salt, seasoned salt, or sugar, and roast for 45 to 50 minutes in a 325°F oven.

YELLOW VEGETABLES

CORN, SCALLIONS, & TOMATOES
With this recipe, you can have the taste of late summer year-round

If you make this dish during the summer when young sweet corn is available, it's wonderful. However, you can use frozen or canned corn during the winter and create almost the same effect. Cherry tomatoes and fresh basil are available year-round, but you can substitute dried basil if necessary.

Spice up the tomatoes with cayenne pepper, adjusting the heat to your family's taste buds. Use fresh or dried rosemary with the basil or marjoram. Sage leaves are also quite good with this, giving the dish a totally different flavor.

This colorful meal is very attractive when served in a rustic terra-cotta or ceramic dish. *Yield: 4 servings*

Ingredients

4 ears young corn, shucked (if the corn is mature, it must be precooked)

$1/2$ cup low-fat margarine

1 bunch scallions, chopped

1 bunch basil leaves, rinsed and chopped, or other herbs, fresh or dried

1 teaspoon dried thyme or 1 teaspoon dried rosemary (optional)

Salt and freshly ground black pepper to taste

1 pint cherry tomatoes, rinsed, halved, and roasted

Calories 105, **Fat** (g) 2, **Carbohydrates** (g) 22, **Protein** (g) 4, **Fiber** (g) 4, **Saturated Fat** (g) 1, **Cholesterol** (mg) 0, **Sodium** (mg) 187, **Carb Choice** 1, **ADA Exchange** 1 starch, 1 vegetable

Corn, Scallions, & Tomatoes

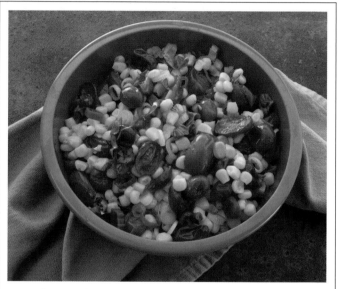

- Cut the corn from the cob onto a piece of waxed paper.

- In a large sauté pan, melt the margarine; add the corn, and poach for 3 to 4 minutes. Then add scallions, basil, optional herb, salt, and pepper.

- Add roasted tomatoes to the corn and butter mixture. Heat thoroughly.

- Place in a serving dish and enjoy.

Great additions and substitutions: If you add 1 package frozen edamame soybeans, cooked, to the corn and tomatoes, it becomes a classic combination called succotash. This will add 2 servings to your yield. You can also add 1 cup fresh or frozen green baby peas to this recipe. And 1 small jar roasted red peppers; or chipotle peppers add a nice zing.

A main dish for vegetarians: To turn this recipe into a vegetarian entree, add 8 ounces cubed white or orange low-fat cheddar cheese and 1 package frozen lima beans, cooked. Run dish under the broiler to melt cheese. For vegans, who eat absolutely no animal products, add cubes of satin tofu and either 1 package lima beans, cooked, or 1 can black beans to the basic recipe.

Roasting Cherry Tomatoes

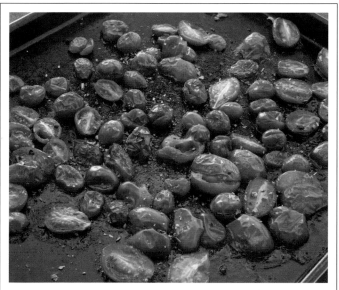

- Preheat the oven to 300°F. Prepare a cookie sheet with aluminum foil and coat with nonstick spray.

- Wash and cut the tomatoes in half. Arrange on the baking sheet and brush them with olive oil.

- Sprinkle the tomatoes, cut side up, with cayenne pepper or freshly ground black pepper.

- You can also sprinkle them with dried oregano and salt as options.

Olive Oil: Brush or Spray?

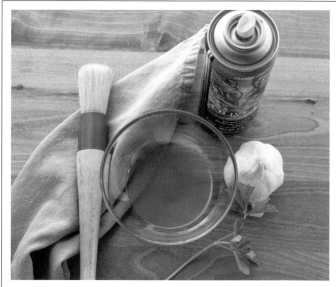

- There are good reasons for brushing and for spraying olive oil. When you spray it, it's generalized and covers a wider area.

- Spray olive oil on salad greens, large vegetables, and bowls of veggies that you plan to eat raw or cooked.

- It's better to brush olive oil onto the cherry tomatoes on the baking sheet to get most of the oil on the tomatoes and less on the sheet.

- Pastry brushes come in several sizes. Use the smallest on the tomatoes.

YELLOW VEGETABLES

ROASTED CAULIFLOWER

Even the pickiest eaters will be surprised at the taste of this unique dish

Cauliflower is exceptionally good for you. It contains zero fat, lots of vitamin C and fiber, and very good carbs, in addition to micronutrients that we all need.

When you roast cauliflower, the natural sugars are concentrated and caramelized, and the cauliflower becomes crispy. You have loads of flavoring options. Parmesan or Romano

cheese is very nice, and aside from salt and pepper, you can use chili powder for spice. This recipe provides a different and healthy alternative to the creamy stuff or plain steamed cauliflower. Although a cauliflower gratin tastes very good, it also contains a lot of fat and calories. This recipe is more in line with the goals of diabetes management. *Yield: 4 servings*

Ingredients

1 head cauliflower, cleaned

2 tablespoons olive oil

1 teaspoon salt

$^1/_2$ teaspoon cayenne pepper or chili powder, or both

Freshly ground black pepper to taste

2 tablespoons Parmesan cheese (optional)

Calories 103, **Fat** (g) 7, **Carbohydrates** (g) 7, **Protein** (g) 3, **Fiber** (g) 4, **Saturated Fat** (g) 2, **Cholesterol** (mg) 0, **Sodium** (mg) 25, **ADA Exchange** 1 vegetable, 1½ fat

Roasted Cauliflower

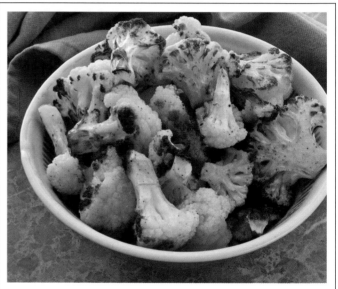

- Preheat oven to 500°F. Remove green leaves and core of the cauliflower. Break into small florets, cutting off long stems. Rinse well; dry thoroughly between paper towels.

- Mix the olive oil, salt, and seasonings in a large bowl.

- Toss the florets in the oil mixture.

- Place florets on a cookie sheet that you have prepared with nonstick spray. Roast at least 30 minutes. Turn cauliflower and continue to roast until deep, golden brown.

Fun variations: Experiment with adding garlic powder, onion powder, and some of the seasonings that are formulated to substitute for salt. Try crushing some caraway seeds with salt for a different and delicious flavoring. While you are at it, roast some carrots whole and serve a medley of veggies. Try making very small florets and serving the cauliflower with toothpicks as a snack, which would be especially nice accompanied by a dipping sauce. Use any good-quality tomato sauce or your own fresh pasta sauce. You might try a low-cal Russian dressing with low-fat mayonnaise, chili sauce, and chopped scallions, or onions and dill pickle.

Cleaning and Preparing Cauliflower

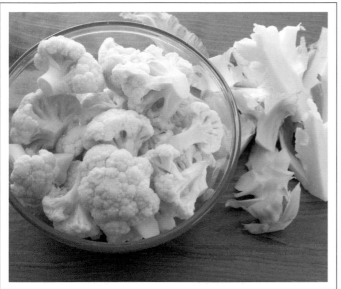

- Pull or cut off the green leaf stems and discard. Cut the cauliflower into quarters.

- Cut out the core and discard it.

- Break the quarters into florets. Make them smaller for snacks and larger for side dishes.

- Rinse the florets under cool running water. Make sure they are dry before adding seasonings and roasting.

Why Dry Cauliflower Before Roasting?

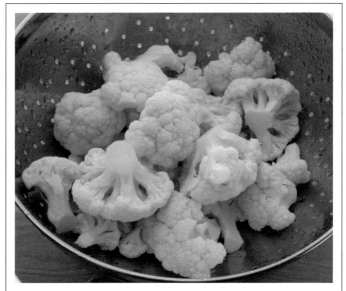

- It's important to dry cauliflower before roasting for a couple of reasons. One, it will get mushy and steam rather than roast if it's still wet.

- Two, the oil and seasonings will drip off wet cauliflower, but they will adhere well to dry cauliflower.

- If you can't get the florets dry between paper towels, let them air-dry for an hour or so.

- Only add the olive oil and seasonings when the cauliflower is dry and ready to go into the oven.

YELLOW VEGETABLES

LENTIL & SAUSAGE CASSEROLE

A little bit of turkey sausage goes a long way in this hearty mix of veggies and lentils

You can mix just about any meat and/or vegetable into a lentil dish, and it will be delicious. If you don't want to use turkey sausage, you can substitute pieces of chicken, pork, or lamb.

This casserole is very easy to make. Lentils come in a variety of colors. The gray-green ones are the most prevalent and readily available. There are also smaller French ones, as well as red, orange, and yellow lentils. They all provide a great source of protein and fiber, particularly for vegetarians who may not be getting other sources of protein in this meal. *Yield: 6 servings*

Ingredients

1 tablespoon olive oil

1 pound turkey sausage, cut into 1-inch pieces

2 large onions, red or white, peeled and cut into chunks

4 cloves garlic, smashed and peeled

2 carrots, peeled and cut into 1-inch pieces

2 parsnips, peeled and cut into 1-inch pieces

2 cups lentils, uncooked and rinsed

3 cups chicken broth or water

Salt and black pepper to taste

Pinch of ground cloves

2 bay leaves

Calories 235, **Fat** (g) 8, **Carbohydrates** (g) 29, **Protein** (g) 14, **Fiber** (g) 9, **Saturated Fat** (g) 3, **Cholesterol** (mg) 30, **Sodium** (mg) 544, **Carb Choices** 2, **ADA Exchange** 2 starch, 1 lean meat, 1 fat

Lentil & Sausage Casserole

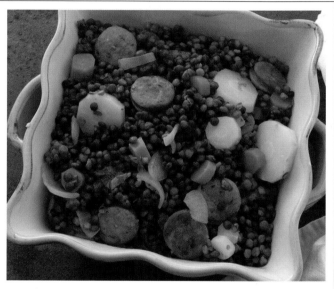

- Preheat oven to 325°F.

- On the stovetop, heat oil in a large, ovenproof casserole dish over medium heat. Lightly brown the sausage, onion, and garlic.

- Add the rest of the ingredients. Cover and place the casserole in the oven; bake for 1 hour.

- Check for doneness by tasting a small spoonful of lentils. If tough, cook longer. Check for doneness every 15 minutes or so.

One of the great things about lentils is that you don't have to soak them prior to cooking. Not only that, they also take far less time to cook than other beans. However, you can use any bean you wish in this recipe, or you can substitute split peas, green or yellow. The easiest option is to use canned beans. Otherwise, you have to soak the beans (other than lentils) for several hours or overnight and cook them for three to four hours. Red or white beans are very good in casseroles, and the canned ones are always softer than those you cook yourself. If you use beans, you can omit the meat, as the beans have a great deal of excellent protein.

Rinse Your Lentils

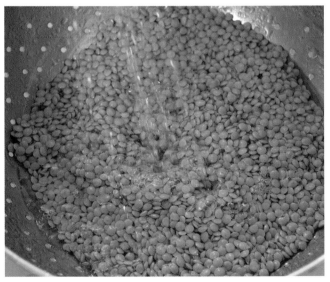

- Always rinse your lentils under cool running water.

- This will melt any lumps of mud they may have acquired in harvesting.

- Rinsing will also make pebbles more visible, as they change color when wet.

- A good rinse will also freshen them up, removing any dust they might have picked up.

Storing Dried Lentils and Beans

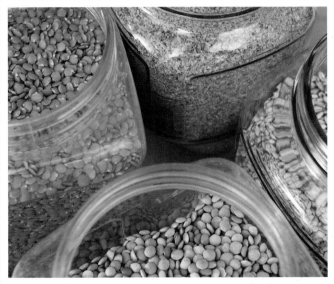

- Dried lentils and other dried beans must be stored in airtight containers; plastic is fine.

- They should not be subjected to dampness, or they will get moldy.

- Beans and lentils should not be kept loose in a bag, or they will attract bugs.

- Mice love to get into bags of beans. Be sure that the container has a tight lid.

WARM LENTIL SALAD

Lentils with roasted sweet red peppers and napa cabbage are a study in contrasting textures and flavors

The texture of the warm lentils is soft; the cabbage is crisp. The lentils have a nutty flavor, and the peppers are sweet.

Napa cabbage may be the most underused of all cabbages, yet it is one of the most versatile. It is good raw or cooked, in combination with other ingredients or on its own. Its pale green color and crunchy texture make it an ideal contrast to the other items in this salad.

You can either roast the red peppers yourself or buy a jar of roasted peppers at the supermarket.

The garnish for this salad is very much to your own taste. Black olives, Greek or Italian, add a sharp touch, as does the recommended vinaigrette. *Yield: 4 servings*

Ingredients

2 cups dried lentils, rinsed

1/2 cup water and 1/2 cup red wine vinegar

4 tablespoons olive oil

1 teaspoon prepared mustard

1 teaspoon Worcestershire sauce

Juice of 1/2 lemon

Salt and pepper to taste

1/2 cup sweet roasted red pepper, diced

4 cups shredded napa cabbage, rinsed and shredded

Optional garnish: 1/2 cup pitted and chopped Greek or Italian olives, 2 tablespoons capers, or 1 tablespoon green peppercorns

Calories 359, **Fat** (g) 19, **Carbohydrates** (g) 33, **Protein** (g) 14, **Fiber** (g) 15, **Saturated Fat** (g) 4, **Cholesterol** (mg) 0, **Sodium** (mg) 62, **Carb Choices** 2, **ADA Exchange** 2 starch, 1 medium-fat meat, 2 fat

Warm Lentil Salad

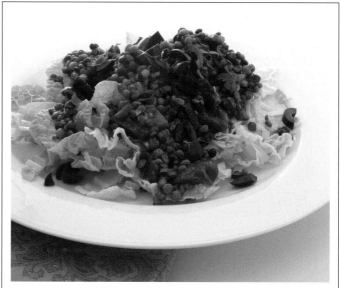

- Over medium heat, cook the lentils in ½ cup vinegar with enough water to cover for 30 minutes.

- In a bowl, whisk together ¼ cup vinegar, olive oil, mustard, Worcestershire sauce, and lemon juice.

- Drain the lentils and place in a large bowl; add the dressing, salt, pepper, and red peppers.

- Divide the cabbage among serving plates. Arrange the lentils over the cabbage, and garnish as desired.

• • • • RECIPE VARIATION • • • •

Some good substitutes: Although napa cabbage is recommended for this dish, you can substitute romaine or iceberg lettuce. Just be sure to use something good and crunchy with a slightly sweet taste. You can use beans other than lentils; however, the lentils hold the flavor of the vinegar, which you add to the cooking liquid, and they have a tangier flavor than beans with thick skins. You can substitute chickpeas, yellow or green split peas, or use any color lentil you wish. However, the small, French gray-green ones seem to come out the best in this recipe. If you decide not to use olives for garnish, add a few capers. For a sophisticated touch, garnish with green peppercorns packed in brine.

Roasting Red Peppers

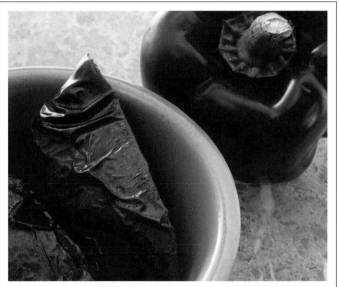

- Roasted red peppers are sensational in salads and soups, and as garnishes and hors d'oeuvres.

- If you have a gas stove, put a pepper on a long-handled metal fork and hold it over the flame, turning until evenly charred.

- Or, cut peppers in half and remove the seeds and cores. Place on greased aluminum foil under a preheated gas or electric broiler.

- To remove charred skin, place in a plastic bag right after cooking. When cooled, the skins will slip right off.

Precooking Lentils for Salad

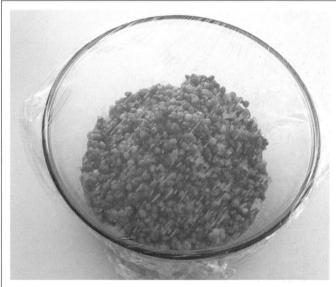

- To enhance the flavor of lentils for salads, cook them the day or night before. Then marinate them in the dressing suggested for the recipe.

- Use any vinaigrette, with vinegar, or make a citrus dressing. Just use plenty of flavorings, herbs, and garlic.

- Be sure the lentils are well coated with dressing.

- Dress the lentils in a nonreactive bowl—glass or ceramic is best. Cover tightly and marinate overnight.

CANNELLINI BEANS & DUCK

Adding aromatic vegetables to this lovely dish makes it an ideal winter entrée

A take-off on cassoulet, a complex French casserole, this recipe is not nearly as difficult or time-consuming as the classic, and it's delicious.

If you can't get duck breasts, substitute pork tenderloin. However, your meat market should be able to order frozen duck breasts for you, or you can get them online. Keep in mind that duck is much higher in total fat and saturated fat than other poultry. It is fine to have occasionally, though. Using canned beans is a huge time-saver. Sausage is an optional addition to this dish and adds flavor and volume. Fresh thyme is another excellent flavor important to this dish. Use dried thyme if you can't find fresh. *Yield: 6 servings*

Ingredients

1 tablespoon flour

Sprinkling of salt and pepper

2 duck breasts, about ⅓ pound each, thawed if frozen, or 1 pork tenderloin, about 10 to 12 ounces

2 tablespoons olive oil

½ pound Italian or Polish turkey sausage, cut into chunks

1 cup yellow, white, or red sweet onions, chopped

4 cloves garlic, smashed and peeled

3 carrots, peeled and chopped

3 parsnips, peeled and chopped

3 stalks celery, cut into bite-size pieces

1 celery root (celeriac), peeled and cut into small pieces

1 cup chicken broth

1 cup canned Italian plum tomatoes, drained and chopped

1 tablespoon dried or 4 teaspoons fresh rosemary or thyme

2 13-ounce cans cannellini beans, drained and rinsed

⅓ cup fresh bread crumbs or 2 tablespoons dried bread crumbs

Calories 369, **Fat** (g) 13, **Carbohydrates** (g) 47, **Protein** (g) 18, **Fiber** (g) 14, **Saturated Fat** (g) 4, **Cholesterol** (mg) 29, **Sodium** (mg) 931, **Carb Choices** 3, **ADA Exchange** 2 starch, 3 nonstarchy vegetable, 1 high-fat meat, 1 fat

Cannellini Beans with Duck

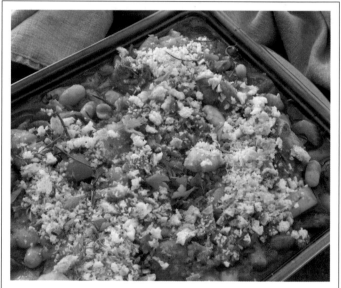

- Preheat oven to 350°F. Sprinkle flour, salt, and pepper on waxed paper. Roll duck (or pork) in flour mixture. On top of stove, heat olive oil in large, ovenproof casserole.

- Brown duck and sausage; remove from pan. Sauté onion, garlic, carrots, parsnips, celery, and celery root in casserole.

- Add broth, tomatoes, herbs, beans. Cut sausage and duck (or pork) into pieces. Return meat to casserole.

- Mix well; sprinkle with bread crumbs. Bake 45 minutes. Serve.

• • • • RECIPE VARIATION • • • •

Good substitutions: You can use Italian-style sausage or kielbasa (Polish sausage) in this dish, if you opt to add sausage. A half pound of sausage will add two to three servings to the yield. You can also substitute rosemary for thyme. Rosemary works very well with duck, chicken, pork, or turkey. It is a terrific aromatic herb that also goes beautifully with lamb.

Party-size proportions: For a party, double the recipe and serve it buffet-style. On the side, have plenty of multigrain French or Italian bread, toasted and drizzled with a little olive oil and a sprinkling of herbs. A big green salad with lots of romaine lettuce and arugula, watercress, or baby spinach also goes very well with this casserole.

Brown and De-fat Your Sausage

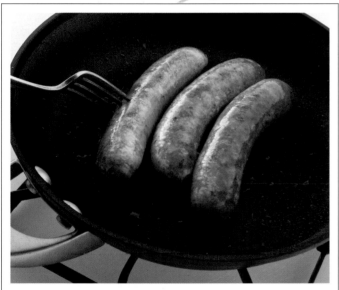

Party Dishes: Bite-size Pieces

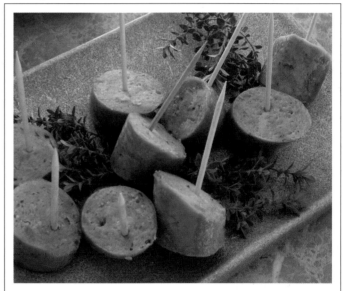

- When you brown sausage before using it in any dish, try to get most of the fat out of it.

- Of course, if you are using turkey sausage, you probably won't have a lot of fat. However, pork and beef sausage may be quite fatty.

- When heated, the fat liquefies. Thus, if you prick the sausage with a fork, the fat will run out into the pan.

- Then you can drain off the fat, leaving just enough oil for your vegetables.

- For a buffet-style party, it's important to have all your ingredients in bite-size pieces for your guests.

- With little effort, you can cut up your meat and vegetables, and tear or shred your salad.

- The last thing you want is guests dropping half of their dinner in their laps or on the floor.

- Think ahead, and prepare your party dishes early so that you have plenty of time for chopping and cutting the ingredients.

125

CANNELLINI BEANS & MEATBALLS

A pot of cannellini beans can serve as a great base for meats, eggplant, and seasonings

Tiny meatballs are an Italian favorite. They are an essential ingredient in Italian wedding soup, which also contains beans, pasta, and vegetables.

Make lots of meatballs, and store them in the freezer. Then, if guests pop in unexpectedly, you can use them for cocktail snacks, or add them to some pasta sauce and feed a crowd.

Using ground turkey saves lots of calories, and meatballs have an excellent flavor when well seasoned. Picky eaters love these treats. They are great for portion control. A few meatballs go a long way when served with beans and vegetables. Shredded carrots, chopped tomatoes, zucchini, and peas are also good in this dish. *Yield: 4 servings*

Ingredients

¹/₂ pound ground turkey (used for analysis), veal, or lean beef

¹/₂ cup soft bread crumbs

1 tablespoon chili sauce

1 tablespoon milk

1 clove garlic, minced

1 teaspoon onion powder

1 teaspoon oregano

Salt and freshly ground black pepper to taste

Pinch of cinnamon

1 egg

1 tablespoon olive oil

1 large onion, peeled and chopped

3 cloves garlic, peeled and chopped

1¹/₂ cups well-seasoned tomato sauce

2 13-ounce cans cannellini beans, drained and rinsed

¹/₂ cup chicken or beef broth

Calories 383, **Fat** (g) 5, **Carbohydrates** (g) 60, **Protein** (g) 27, **Fiber** (g) 13, **Saturated Fat** (g) 1, **Cholesterol** (mg) 26, **Sodium** (mg) 719, **Carb Choices** 3½, **ADA Exchange** 4 starch, 2 very lean meat

Cannellini Beans & Meatballs

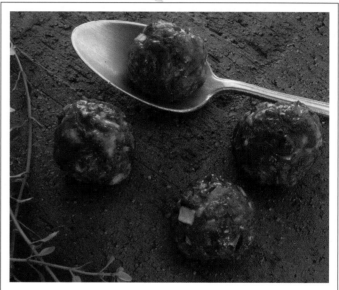

- Preheat oven to 325°F. Mix the first 10 ingredients in a bowl. Form into very small meatballs (about 1 inch in diameter).

- Place onto a baking sheet that you've prepared with nonstick spray. Bake for 25 minutes. When done, drain on paper towels.

- Heat olive oil in a large pot. Sauté onion and garlic over medium heat until softened.

- Add tomato sauce, beans, broth, and meatballs. Stir gently so as not to break up meatballs but rather cover them completely with sauce.

If you are watching your budget, beans are an excellent source of nutrition and a fine way to stretch a dollar. They can also serve as a meat substitute, adding protein and fiber to a meal. Beans by themselves are bland in flavor and need plenty of aromatic vegetables and herbs.

• • • • RECIPE VARIATION • • • •

Lower-calorie meatballs: Make meatballs with ground veal or lean ground beef. Because ground turkey has less fat and fewer calories, it is preferable. Dried cannellini beans are terrific; however, they must be soaked—overnight is best. If you cook beans and vegetables together, making a gravy while you prepare meatballs, the results are delicious. The beans soak up the flavors.

Using a Melon Ball Scoop

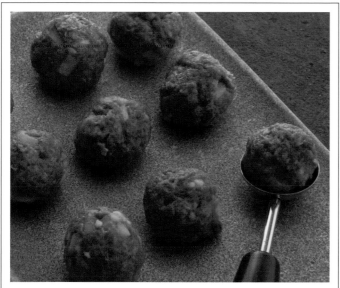

Adding Spices to Ground Meats

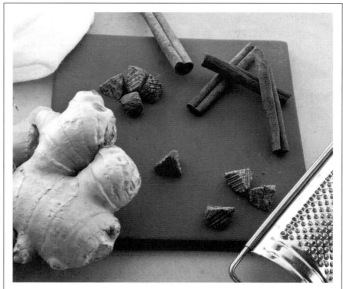

- Use a melon ball scoop to form your meatballs evenly.

- Or, use a teaspoon. Just be sure to roll the balls between your palms to compress them and make them round. Elliptical meatballs, shaped like footballs, do not brown evenly.

- If meatballs are all the same size, they should cook evenly.

- If the meatballs are not baking evenly because your oven does not provide even heat, turn the pan and roll the balls over from time to time.

- It's an Italian tradition to put a pinch of cinnamon in meatballs and meat sauce.

- A pinch is $\frac{1}{16}$ to $\frac{1}{8}$ teaspoon. You don't want to use enough to make the flavor pronounced, or even barely discernible. What you want to achieve is a delightful hint.

- You can also use fresh or candied ginger in turkey, pork, and beef dishes.

- When fresh ginger was unavailable, cooks would crumble gingersnaps into beef stew, adding enough zip to make the stew interesting.

TURKEY CHILI WITH BEANS

Quick to make and perfect for a crowd, this chili is high in flavor but low in fat

The longer you cook chili, the better it is. You can use a slow cooker and start the cooking before you go to bed at night, or early in the morning before you go to work or your child's ball game. Just let the slow cooker do its thing.

If you don't have a slow cooker, you must be very careful to set your stove on simmer so that the chili won't burn. Burned chili is ruined chili—it can't be saved. Or, bake the chili in your oven, set on 250°F for three to six hours. The various seasonings make this chili different. You will find your guests licking their lips and asking about that delicious flavor. Of course, it's many flavors married together and an unusual secret ingredient—cocoa powder. *Yield: 10 servings*

Ingredients

¹/₄ cup olive or canola oil

1 pound ground turkey

4 yellow cooking onions, peeled and coarsely chopped

4 cloves garlic, smashed and chopped

3 sweet green peppers, cored, seeded, and diced

1–2 serrano peppers, or 3 jalapeño peppers, chopped, seeds in for exra heat

1 sweet red pepper, cored, seeded, roasted and peeled, (from a jar is fine)

2 teaspoons unsweetened cocoa powder

2 teaspoons dried thyme leaves

2 tablespoons chili powder, or to taste

1 teaspoon freshly ground black pepper

1 teaspoon salt

¹/₂ can (about 6 ounces) low-sodium beef broth

1 28-ounce can Italian plum tomatoes

6 ounces flat beer

1 pound red kidney beans, soaked overnight* (used for analysis), or 4 cans red kidney beans, drained and rinsed

*If you use dried beans, you will need more water.

Calories 344, **Fat** (g) 11, **Carbohydrates** (g) 42, **Protein** (g) 22, **Fiber** (g) 13, **Saturated Fat** (g) 3, **Cholesterol** (mg) 37, **Sodium** (mg) 180, **Carb Choices** 2½, **ADA Exchange** 2½ starch, 2½ medium-fat meat

Turkey Chili with Beans

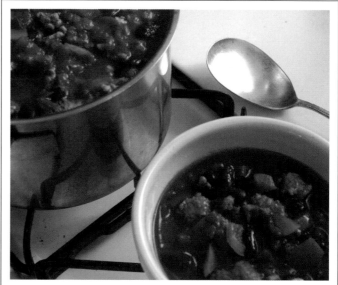

- Heat the olive oil in a large pot and lightly brown the turkey, then add the vegetables. Cook until the onions are transparent.

- Stir in the cocoa powder, thyme, chili powder, pepper, and salt; mix well.

- Add the liquids, tomatoes, and beans; stir to blend. Pour into slow cooker and cook on low for 4 to 6 hours. Or bake in the oven at 250°F for at least 3 to 4 hours.

Seasoning your chili: Some of the flavorings in this recipe will surprise you. Cocoa, an ancient Inca flavoring, charms the palate without overwhelming the integrity of the chili. You will also add ½ bottle of good beer—Mexican beer is great. I like using Italian tomatoes that come in a box—they have a fresher taste than the canned ones. A good chili powder is a must, as are some fresh and canned chipotle chilies—and don't forget sweet peppers. Add red pepper flakes if you don't have time to prepare fresh hot chilies. For a leaner option, turkey replaces beef very nicely. Many chili contests have been won using ground turkey. However, if you do use beef, choose lean chuck (more than 90 percent lean, or fat-free), ground coarsely.

Checking Your Beans for Doneness

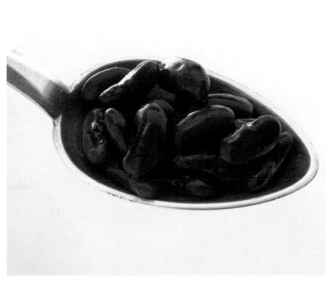

- Beans that have not cooked enough are not very good to eat. They are hard, dry, and tasteless.

- If you are using dried beans, they may require 1 cup more liquid from time to time, even though you've soaked them.

- Make sure they don't dry out. Add more beer, broth, or water to keep them nice and saucy.

- When you are checking your beans for doneness, also check the flavoring. Adjust for salt and add spice.

Fire-Roasted Chili

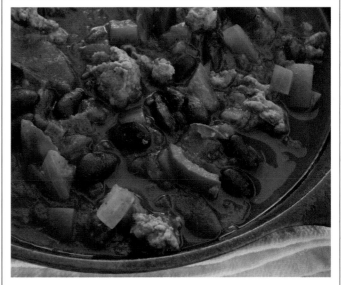

- Many chili recipes call for roasting chili over a wood fire.

- You can do this under your broiler or over a gas flame on the stovetop.

- Place the final chili ingredients in a cast-iron pot over a low, smoky fire. Do not cover for 3 hours. Or bake in the oven at 250°F for 3 hours.

PINK BEANS, MAC, & KALE
This dish shines with flavor when kale is in season

The minute you see huge bunches of fresh kale, dark green and crisp, in the supermarket, buy it. Kale is a fantastic vegetable that is incredibly nutritious, as it is filled with antioxidants.

When you buy kale, there should be no limp, yellow, or "tired"-looking leaves. The whole bunch should epitomize freshness.

When you get it home, remove the heavy stems all the way up to the leaves. Discard the stems. Break it up, and then run the kale under cool water to remove sand and grit.

When perfectly clean, drain and wrap the kale in a clean dish towel or paper towels. Place in a plastic bag and refrigerate until ready to use. *Yield: 6 servings*

Ingredients

2 tablespoons olive oil

1 cup sweet onions, chopped

2 cloves garlic, peeled and chopped

2 tablespoons tomato paste

2 cups chicken or vegetable broth

1 large bunch kale, stemmed, cleaned, and torn into pieces

2 cups pasta

2 13-ounce cans pink beans, drained and rinsed

1 tablespoon dried rosemary

1 teaspoon dried oregano

Salt and pepper to taste

Garnish: 6 half-teaspoons grated Parmesan cheese, freshly chopped parsley

Calories 236, **Fat** (g) 6, **Carbohydrates** (g) 37, **Protein** (g) 11, **Fiber** (g) 5, **Saturated Fat** (g) 1, **Cholesterol** (mg) 1, **Sodium** (mg) 215, **Carb Choices** 2½, **ADA Exchange** 2½ starch

Pink Beans, Mac, & Kale

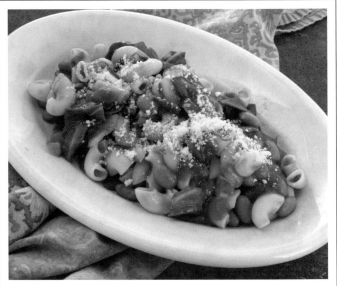

- Heat oil in a large pot. Add onions and garlic; sauté until soft, about 4 to 5 minutes.

- Stir in tomato paste and broth, then stir in kale. It will fill the pot, but it cooks down. Reduce heat to low; cover and simmer 30 minutes or until kale is tender.

- While the kale cooks, boil the pasta in a pot of lightly salted water. When al dente, drain the pasta.

- Add the cooked pasta and the remaining ingredients to the large pot; cover. Simmer 20 minutes. Serve in individual bowls, garnished as desired.

• • • • RECIPE VARIATION • • • •

Use what you have: This recipe is a variation on the theme of pasta, beans, and vegetables. You can add various meats for flavor. Tiny shell macaroni or other small pasta makes a good substitute for elbows. Orecchiette, pasta in the shape of small ears, tastes wonderful in this dish and is fun, too. Or use rigatoni or curly noodles. The sweetness of the beans is accented by the somewhat sharp flavor of the kale, but this dish is also very good when made with fresh escarole. Other vegetables to add into this recipe include carrots, celery, parsnips, baby blue nose turnips, and yellow beets, all cut into a small dice. Red beets turn everything too red , so save them for another dish.

Cooking Down Greens

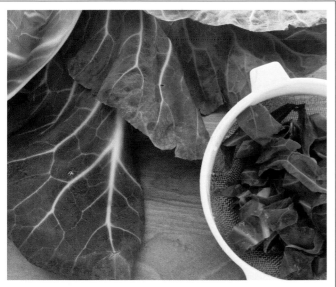

- You may think that your huge bunch of kale, collards, or turnip greens will feed at least ten people.

- But after you cook enough greens to fill a gallon pot, you end up with barely enough for four.

- When you cook them on the stovetop, the greens will greatly shrink and condense.

- Before you cook down the greens, you should remove the stems, which are tough and woody and often aren't good for soup.

Soaking Beans

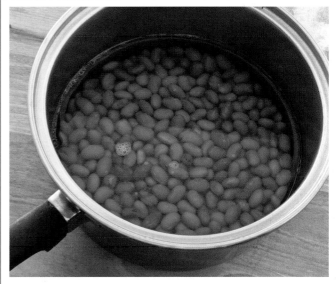

- Some beans require less soaking time than others. Lentils do not need to be soaked at all.

- Beans with stronger shells—such as lima, red or white kidney, and pinto—require an overnight soak.

- Some cooks bring the white, red, and pink beans to a boil in a pot with enough water to cover them. Then, they turn off the heat, cover, and soak for 1 hour.

- This may not work so well. You may get lots of tough bean shells. It's better to use canned.

THANKSGIVING TURKEY MEAT LOAF

An excellent meal for both small family get-togethers and large, festive holiday parties

When you want to do something easy that's sure to please, try this recipe for a festive family dinner. You can make it a couple of days in advance and refrigerate the meat loaf, or make it weeks in advance and freeze it.

The cranberries and nuts add interest, fiber, and nutrients. There is vitamin C in orange juice and omega-3 fatty acids in walnuts. If you use dark meat for the ground turkey, the meat loaf will have more flavor than if you use all white meat.

Turkey meat loaf is lighter in calories than beef, pork, or combination meat loaf. You will find that the taste is just as good and the texture appealing if you use plenty of bread crumbs—not dried, but fresh. *Yield: 8 servings*

Ingredients

2 whole eggs

¼ cup milk

¼ cup orange juice

Salt and freshly ground black pepper to taste

1 teaspoon dried thyme leaves

2 teaspoons dried rosemary leaves, crumbled

1½ cups fresh bread crumbs

1¼ pound ground turkey breast

2 tablespoons low-fat margarine

1½ cups celery, minced

½ cup sweet onions, minced

1 cup walnut pieces, toasted

½ cup dried cranberries

Calories 286, **Fat** (g) 14, **Carbohydrates** (g) 21, **Protein** (g) 20, **Fiber** (g) 2, **Saturated Fat** (g) 4, **Cholesterol** (mg) 116, **Sodium** (mg) 338, **Carb Choices** 1½, **ADA Exchange** 1½ starch, 3 medium-fat meat, 1 fat

Thanksgiving Turkey Meat Loaf

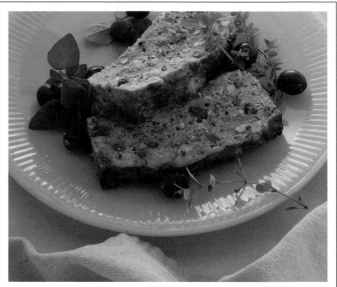

- Preheat oven to 350°F. Whisk together eggs, milk, orange juice, salt, pepper, and herbs in a large mixing bowl. Add bread crumbs and turkey, mixing well.

- Melt margarine in a frying pan; add celery and onion. Sauté until soft, about 5 minutes.

- Add celery-onion mixture to meat, then add walnuts and cranberries. Mix well. Prepare a bread pan (4 x 8 inches) with nonstick spray. Pour meat mixture into pan, spreading evenly.

- Bake 90 minutes. Cool slightly before turning out and cutting into slices.

Fun variations: Turn this into a springtime recipe with a sprinkling of chopped basil and chives and the addition of a box of frozen baby green peas, thawed. Make your meat loaf with a south of the border tang by adding ½ cup salsa and ¼ cup chopped hot chilies, and corn bread crumbs in place of regular bread crumbs. Top this spicy loaf with a dollop of low-fat or fat-free sour cream. A little minced chorizo and roasted red peppers add Spanish flavor, especially if you garnish the finished dish with chopped olives. For an Italian touch, use oregano, basil, and extra garlic to season the loaf. Add ½ cup of a good Italian marinara sauce to the recipe; ½ cup Parmesan cheese enhances the Italian flavorings even more. To lighten loaf, use 2 well-beaten egg whites.

Fluffing Your Mixture

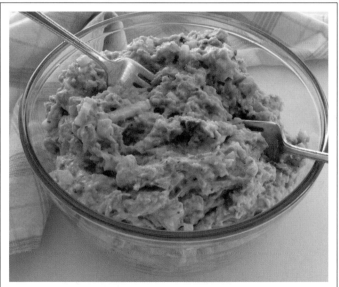

- There are many ways to incorporate ingredients, such as mixing, folding, blending, and fluffing.

- To fluff, place most of the ingredients in a large bowl; the bigger, the better.

- Using two forks, bring the ingredients from the outside of the bowl toward the center. Work your way around the outside of the bowl.

- Add the rest of the ingredients and continue to fluff them up. The result is juicy, not heavily compressed and superdense, meat loaf.

Steaming Meat Loaf in a Bain Marie

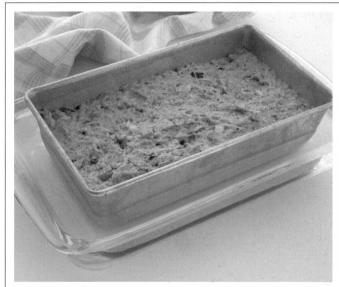

- This technique makes an extremely tender, juicy meat loaf. A bain marie is basically a hot-water bath in the oven.

- Fill a large pan a quarter way up with hot water and place in the oven at 350°F.

- Put the loaf pan containing the meat loaf into the larger pan, and cook according to directions.

- If you need to add water for more steam, add it from a kettle, making sure not to get water on the meat loaf.

BEEF STEW WITH ARTICHOKES

Elevate a basic stew to new heights with the addition of artichokes, canned or frozen

When you add a can or box of artichokes to a beef, veal, or chicken stew, you will have something very different and most elegant.

Artichokes take the "basic" out of basic beef stew. And if you don't want to use canned unmarinated artichokes, use frozen baby artichoke hearts, defrosted and cut in halves. There is a chemical in the artichoke that changes the flavors to something sweetly different.

Artichokes have phytochemicals and vitamins E and C. They are high in fiber and low in calories. They are only fattening when dipped in butter, mayo, or an olive oil and lemon mixture. Eat them plain or with lemon juice. *Yield: 6 servings*

Ingredients

$^1/_4$ cup all-purpose flour

$^1/_2$ teaspoon salt

$^1/_4$ teaspoon freshly ground black pepper

2 pounds lean beef stew meat, cut into cubes

1 tablespoon olive oil

2 onions, peeled and coarsely chopped

2 cloves garlic, peeled and coarsely chopped

$^1/_2$ cup beef broth (canned is fine)

$^1/_2$ cup dry red wine

Zest and juice of $^1/_2$ fresh lemon

1 12-ounce can artichokes, drained and cut into halves, or 1 package frozen baby artichoke hearts, thawed and cut into halves

Extra black pepper to taste

Additional water, if necessary

Optional: Serve over rice or noodles (not in nutritional analysis)

Calories 338, **Fat** (g) 11, **Carbohydrates** (g) 13, **Protein** (g) 42, **Fiber** (g) 3, **Saturated Fat** (g) 4, **Cholesterol** (mg) 82, **Sodium** (mg) 490, **Carb Choice** 1, **ADA Exchange** 1 starch, 8½ very lean meat

Beef Stew with Artichokes

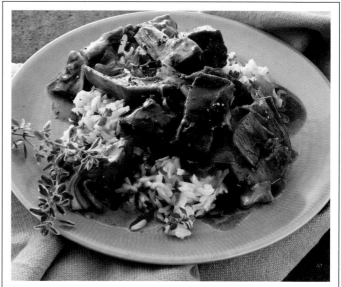

- Mix flour, salt, and pepper on a piece of waxed paper. Roll beef into the flour mixture and set aside.

- Heat oil in a stew pot. Add beef and sauté over medium heat. Reduce heat; move meat to side of pan. Add onions and garlic; cook until soft, about 5 minutes.

- Add remaining ingredients; cover and reduce heat. Simmer until meat is tender, about 2 to 3 hours. Check occasionally, adding more water, wine, or broth if the stew becomes too dry.

- Serve over noodles or brown rice (optional).

Hungarian-style goulash: This basic recipe can quickly become Hungarian-style goulash. When you start the stew, add 1 cup tomato sauce or 1 cup drained plum tomatoes. Add 3 bay leaves and a few drops of Worcestershire sauce. Sprinkle with 1 teaspoon caraway seeds and 1 tablespoon sweet paprika; mix in 2 cups chopped baby carrots. Just before serving the goulash, add 1 cup low-fat sour cream and mix into the gravy, or top each serving with its own dollop of sour cream. If you've made a double recipe for serving later, it's best to add the sour cream individually to each serving. Stew kept in the refrigerator or freezer is much better off without the sour cream, which can separate in the stew over time.

Remove Bay Leaves Before Serving

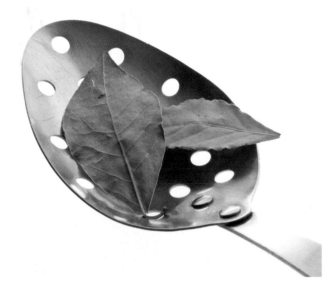

- Bay leaves add a lot of flavor to soups and stews; however, they also pose some dangers.

- Bay leaves are hard and indigestible. They also have sharp edges and can actually cut the esophagus and the lining of the stomach.

- Dried bay leaves are only sold in powdered form in Europe.

- Cooks working with fresh leaves must be sure to remove them before serving soups and stews. Or warn guests to remove them before eating.

Meat for Stew

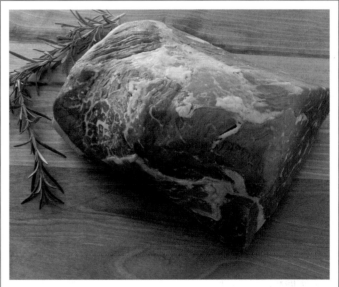

- Because of the long cooking time, you can use a very inexpensive cut of meat to make stews and soups.

- Chuck is flavorful, and once it is cut up and stewed, it will be tender. Round is lower in fat than chuck, so if cutting fat is a priority, choose round.

- Rump or bottom-round roasts are also very good in stews.

- Many cuts are available for stews and soups. Different regions have different names for them. When in doubt, ask the butcher.

THAI CHICKEN TENDERS

Americans are discovering, and falling in love with, spicy Thai food

Thai food can be very spicy—hot is the true adjective. Although this recipe has some heat, it is adjustable for those who have sensitive palates.

Chicken tenders are available fresh and frozen. A big bag of them, stored in the freezer, is a boon for the cook in a rush. Chicken tenders make it easy to prepare a healthy, low-carb, low-calorie meal.

A bit of coconut milk adds creamy sweetness, but use only a tiny amount, as in this recipe. Note that the milk adds saturated fat, so you may want to omit it. Red or green chili paste is available at Asian markets and online, and most supermarkets carry Asian sesame seed oil. Instead of Asian fish sauce, you can use Worcestershire sauce for added flavor. *Yield: 6 servings*

Ingredients

¹/₄ cup all-purpose flour

¹/₂ teaspoon salt

1¹/₂ pounds chicken tenders, cut crosswise into thin strips

1 tablespoon peanut oil, plus 1 tablespoon to use with veggies

1 teaspoon Asian sesame seed oil

4 scallions, chopped

2 cups napa cabbage, shredded

1 teaspoon cornstarch

3 ounces unsweetened coconut milk

¹/₃ cup chicken broth

1 teaspoon green or red Thai chili paste

Salt to taste

2 tablespoons chopped cilantro or parsley

Garnish: ¹/₄ cup unsalted roasted peanuts

Calories 280, **Fat** (g) 14, **Carbohydrates** (g) 9, **Protein** (g) 30, **Fiber** (g) 1, **Saturated Fat** (g) 5, **Cholesterol** (mg) 73, **Sodium** (mg) 294, **Carb Choice** ½, **ADA Exchange** ½ starch, 5 lean meat

Thai Chicken Tenders

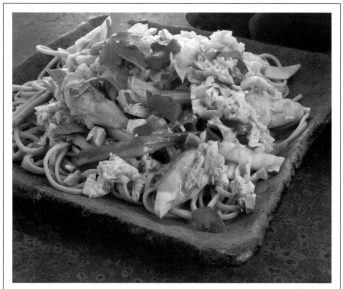

- Spread flour and salt on waxed paper; dredge chicken strips in flour. Heat 1 tablespoon peanut and sesame oils in a sauté pan or wok. Sauté chicken strips on medium-high heat, turning until golden brown on both sides. Remove cooked chicken and set aside.

- Add second tablespoon of oil; sauté scallions and cabbage until crisp-tender, 3 minutes. Place in a bowl. Whisk cornstarch, coconut milk, chicken broth, chili paste in a small bowl; blend into oil left in pan. Fold chicken and vegetables into sauce. Add cilantro and sprinkle with peanuts.

• • • • RECIPE VARIATION • • • •

Improving upon tradition: Traditionally, this recipe would be served with white rice. However, if you are trying to avoid refined and processed carbs in white rice, use brown rice. Oriental noodles are delightful, especially the "glass" or "cellophane" types. Try using whole-grain instead of white noodles. An occasional lapse into true Oriental noodles is not fattening, as the noodles do not include eggs. You can always substitute parsley for cilantro. Peanuts and sauces made with peanut butter are also a staple of Thai cooking.

The Beauties of Stir-Frying

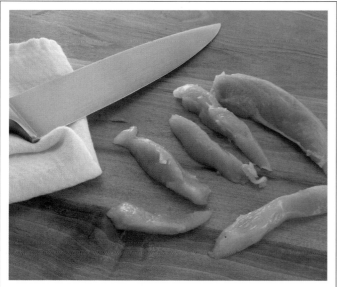

- Because food is cut into small, thin strips, it cooks very quickly when stir-frying.

- Very sharp knives are crucial to creating a successful stir-fry. It's important that all the pieces of meat are almost exactly the same size for even cooking.

- The last thing you want with a stir-fry is to have some of the meat rare and other pieces well done.

- Chicken should never be served rare because it can carry salmonella, a very harmful bacteria.

Shredding Cabbage in a Food Processor

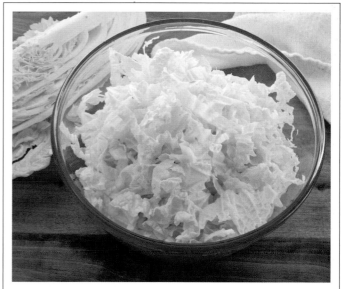

- It's easy to shred cabbage in a food processor. Remove the core and outside leaves. Cut the cabbage lengthwise so that it fits into the tube of the processor.

- Attach the shredding blade. Push the cabbage through with the pusher that comes with the machine.

- Food processors make very short work of shredding cabbage, zucchini, carrots, and just about anything else.

- Using a knife requires a lot more skill and time. Box graters also work well, but be careful of your fingertips.

PISTACHIO-PEPPER STRIP STEAK

Strip steak is terrific served plain, but it's even better with a great crust

Black pepper–crusted steak (steak au poivre) is a traditional French method for preparing filet mignon. It takes advantage of all the flavors that are sealed in by the pepper crust, plus there's a lot of flavor in the pepper itself.

For this recipe, get roasted pistachios that are not salted, if possible. They are available, but you may have to ask for them. If you can't find pistachios, go for hazelnuts (filberts) or cashews.

You can add a drop of brandy to the sauce. Coarse salt crusts on meat or fish are popular with some chefs—they make an igloo out of the salt, and then scrape it off after cooking. *Yield: 6 servings*

Ingredients

²/₃ cup shelled pistachio nuts, coarsely chopped

1 tablespoon black pepper, coarsely ground

¹/₂ teaspoon salt

4 strip steaks, well trimmed, about 6 ounces each

1 tablespoon canola or olive oil

Calories 343, **Fat** (g) 22, **Carbohydrates** (g) 4, **Protein** (g) 31, **Fiber** (g) 2, **Saturated Fat** (g) 7, **Cholesterol** (mg) 70, **Sodium** (mg) 267, **ADA Exchange** 5 medium-fat meat

Pistachio-Pepper Strip Steak

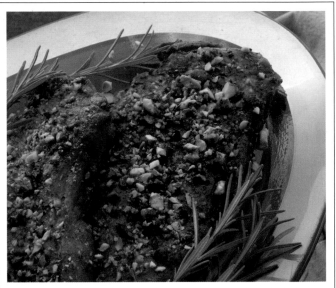

- Evenly spread the nuts, pepper, and salt onto a piece of waxed paper.

- One at a time, place the steaks on the paper, and press the nut mixture into both sides of each steak.

- Heat a sauté pan over medium-high heat. Add the oil. Sauté the steaks 1 minute.

- Turn and reduce heat. Cook over medium-low heat, covered, until desired level of doneness. Let steaks rest for 5 minutes, covered, before serving.

Make it easy and healthful: The best way to prepare this wonderful strip steak is in a sauté pan on top of the stove. Of course, you can put it under the broiler or on the grill, but sautéing both browns the nuts and seals in the flavors. Sautéing is also a very healthful technique when you use canola or olive oil—no butter, please. However, the nuts do produce a buttery flavor when browned with the steak. The nice thing about strip steak is that you can cut off every bit of fat, and it will still be delicious. Also, strip steak is tender enough that you won't need to marinate it or pound it thin to break down the fibers.

When Is Steak Done?

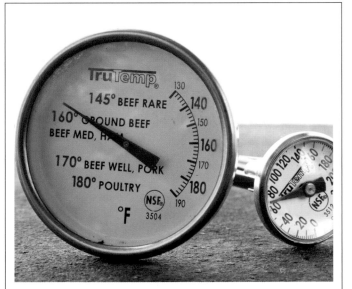

- There are two ways to know if your meat is done.

- First, you can carefully time steaks and roasts. However, because oven temperatures vary greatly, timing can be unreliable.

- Second, you can use a meat thermometer to measure the temperature. Depending on the model, the thermometer will give a reading that will let you know the meat is done.

- A rare steak should be about 135°F; medium, 145°F; and well done, 150°F. Remember, it continues to cook while resting.

Why Let Meat Rest?

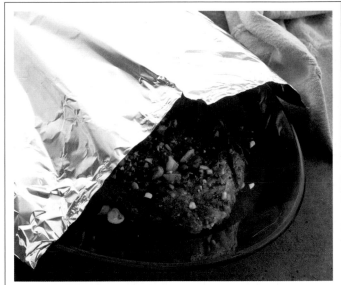

- There are two good reasons for letting a piece of cooked meat rest before cutting into it.

- The first is to let it finish cooking evenly, especially in the center. The second is to make sure the juices do not run out onto the cutting board rather than going back into the meat.

- This principle applies to steaks, roasted turkey, chicken, lamb, beef, and pork.

GRILLED ASIAN CHICKEN THIGHS
These are great snacks for picnics, buffets, and tailgate parties

Your crowd may be a bit tired of Buffalo wings. Try using small thighs, either bone-in or boneless, for a welcome, tasty change. Bone-in is easier to eat outdoors.

Thighs are richer in flavor than wings or breast meat. And, as dark meat, they are slightly higher in calories. They also tend to be far less expensive than wings or breasts, so you get a lot of food for your money.

A nice side with this recipe is fresh orange and shaved fennel salad. Or, a salad of great northern beans with Chinese vegetables (bean sprouts, water chestnuts, and snow peas) with red onions goes really well. *Yield: 8 servings (3 pieces each)*

Ingredients

For the thighs:

1 tablespoon Chinese 5-spice powder (available at most supermarkets)

1 cup brown Splenda

1 tablespoon wasabi powder, more or less or to taste

$1/2$ teaspoon salt

Zest of $1/2$ lemon

24 chicken thighs, bone-in, skinless (3 ounces each)

For the sauce:

1 cup freshly squeezed orange juice

1 tablespoon sugar-free orange marmalade

$1/4$ cup light (low-sodium) soy sauce

1 tablespoon freshly grated gingerroot

Calories 304, **Fat** (g) 8, **Carbohydrates** (g) 14, **Protein** (g) 41, **Fiber** (g) 0, **Saturated Fat** (g) 2, **Cholesterol** (mg) 172, **Sodium** (mg) 449, **Carb Choice** 1, **ADA Exchange** 1 fruit, 6 lean meat

Grilled Asian Chicken Thighs

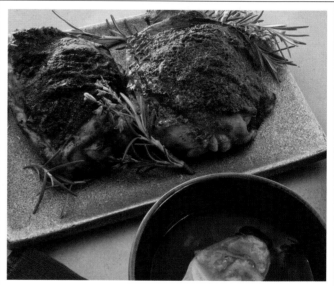

- Place seasonings, lemon zest in a bowl; mix well. Add thighs. Toss to coat well. Work rub under skin of each thigh. Marinate 2 hours or overnight in fridge.

- Prepare grill. Place thighs over medium-high heat 3 minutes; turn and brown 3 minutes more. When thighs are brown on all sides, move them away from direct heat to a cooler part of the grill and close the lid.

- Cook through without burning the thighs, about 7 minutes off to the side.

- Mix sauce items together in a bowl; use for dipping.

Spice rubs and BBQ combinations: You can easily make this recipe for chicken thighs with a Cajun spice rub, or any dry barbecue rub that appeals to you. However, most rubs are high in carbohydrates, so it's best to make your own rubs using brown Splenda. Rubs can also be very high in sodium. A delicious dipping sauce is essential; you can always use salsa, melted cheese, and pepper sauce or, as in this recipe, an Asian/citrus combination. If you use boneless, skinless thighs, you'll find that the spices work themselves into the meat more thoroughly. If using bone-in and skin-on meat, try to work some of the rub under the skin.

Bone-in vs. Boneless Thighs

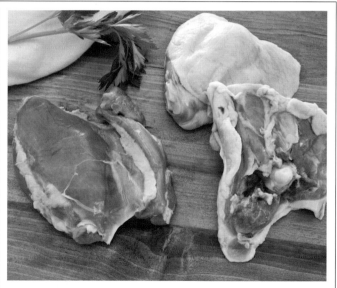

- When using skinless and boneless chicken thighs, you have to be careful not to dry them out. And they are much more difficult to eat out-of-hand than those with bones you can hold on to.

- Thighs with the bone in and skin on take longer to cook, and the skin has more calories.

- Be careful not to burn off the rub, especially when cooking boneless and skinless thighs.

- Cut one piece open to make sure it is done all the way through.

Charcoal vs. Gas

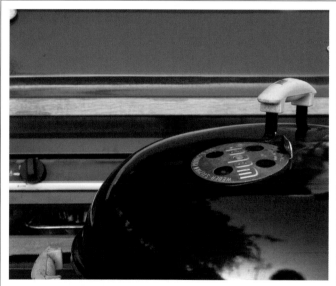

- The flame of a gas grill is easier to control. Some grills even "flash" cook the food at extremely high temperatures.

- A charcoal grill takes longer to bring to the proper temperature. You must let the flames die down and wait until the coals are white.

- Be sure to bank coals to one side so that you can move browned foods away from the direct heat.

- Adding mesquite or other wood chips enhances flavors. A bed of fennel fronds on the rack is also a great addition.

BRAISED VEAL SHANKS

This traditional Italian dish can be a satisfying family dinner or a cozy company meal

Braised veal shanks (*osso bucco*) is a dish for "weekend warriors" in the kitchen, as it takes a fair amount of cooking time.

Veal shanks are thick and have a large marrow bone in the middle. They should have no fat whatsoever on them. You need a big piece, about a half pound per person, because of the bone.

Veal shanks are excellent when served with mashed potatoes, brown rice, or white beans. Pasta, such as orzo, is the traditional Italian accompaniment. Vegetables also go well. You will have lots of sauce when you braise veal shanks. The marrow is wonderful when spread on a thin slice of toasted multigrain bread. *Yield: 6 servings (6-ounce portions)*

Ingredients

2 tablespoons olive oil

6 veal shanks, 2¹/₂ to 3 pounds total weight

Salt and freshly ground black pepper to taste

2 medium-size yellow onions, peeled and chopped

3 cloves garlic, smashed, peeled, and coarsely chopped

¹/₂ cup low-sodium chicken broth

1 cup whole Italian plum tomatoes, drained and chopped

¹/₂ cup dry white wine

2 carrots, peeled and chopped

1 tablespoon dried rosemary

1 teaspoon dried oregano

1 teaspoon dried basil

Garnish: freshly chopped Italian flat-leaf parsley

Calories 337, **Fat** (g) 11, **Carbohydrates** (g) 7, **Protein** (g) 47, **Fiber** (g) 1, **Saturated Fat** (g) 2, **Cholesterol** (mg) 179, **Sodium** (mg) 392, **ADA Exchange** 1 vegetable, 6 lean meat

Braised Veal Shanks

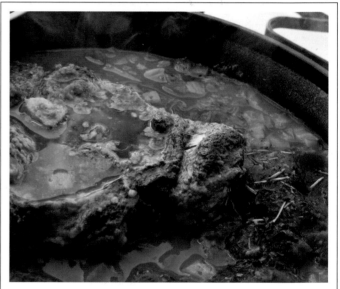

- Heat olive oil over medium-high heat in a Dutch oven or stew pot large enough to hold all of the shanks without crowding.

- Sprinkle veal shanks with salt and pepper; brown them in oil. Remove from pot. Sauté onions and garlic in the pot.

- Add remaining ingredients minus the fresh parsley. Return the shanks to the pan. Cover and reduce heat to simmer. Cook 2 to 3 hours, or until tender.

- Thicken sauce by cooking down or adding a dash of quick-blending flour. Sprinkle with parsley; serve.

Sauces and sides: Veal shanks are delicious in a brown gravy spiked with lemon, and they are also great with mushrooms in a brown sauce. Green olives will make a very good addition; they acquire a rich flavor when cooked. Rosemary, basil, and oregano, together or individually, are fine complements. A side of fennel braised with low-fat margarine and orange slices is also very good.

Salad options: Serve a side salad to add contrast to the veal shanks. If you do not braise fennel as a hot vegetable, you might consider using it shaved, with fresh orange slices and a citrus or white wine vinaigrette. Beet salad with field greens and a bit of goat cheese is also very popular for winter dinners.

Braising Meat

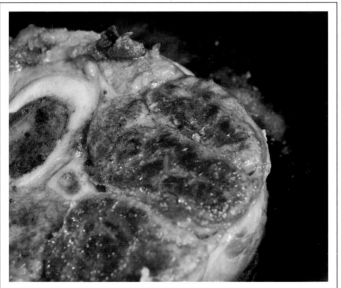

- Braising is a great tenderizer of "muscle" meat. The shank, being part of the leg, is all muscle.

- Beef shanks make great soup. Lamb shanks are excellent when braised.

- To braise, brown meat. Add aromatic vegetables and liquids; reduce heat and cover. Most braising is done on top of the stove, but some put a casserole dish in the oven for 2 to 4 hours, depending on the cut.

- Braising requires very slow cooking until meat is very tender. The cooking liquid becomes sauce or gravy.

Making Gravy and Sauce from Cooking Liquids

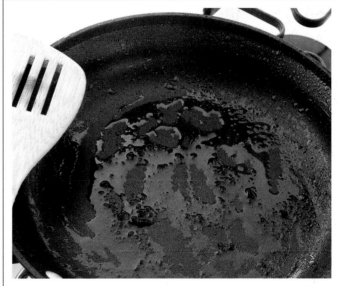

- Once you braise a piece of meat, you should end up with a nice amount of rich juices.

- If you have too much "soup," boil it down to reduce the volume and enrich it.

- Be sure that all of the brown bits on the bottom of the pot dissolve into the sauce. If you don't have enough liquid, add chicken, beef, or vegetable broth and some wine.

- For instant thickening, mix in a sprinkling of quick-blending flour, stirring the gravy/sauce constantly as it comes to a boil.

BROILED HALIBUT WTIH WATERCRESS
Mild and firm with a clean sea flavor, halibut is one of the finest fishes available

Halibut is a huge deep-sea fish. It lives only in clean salt water, and its availability has been declining over the last 20 years because of overfishing.

Halibut doesn't need much in the way of dressing. Too much spicing, dressing, saucing, and/or seasoning masks its natural fresh flavor. Salt, pepper, lemon, and a watercress sauce are all you need. Don't overload with garlic or onions. Bold flavors ruin it. Although firm-fleshed, halibut has a delicate flavor. Flavored bread crumbs moistened with olive oil are good on any fish. With halibut, less is more. Olive oil, used in moderation, is recommended fat that doesn't raise cholesterol. Butter is good melted on fish, and is okay for occasional use. *Yield: 4 servings*

Ingredients

1 tablespoon lemon juice

$^1/_2$ cup chopped watercress

$^1/_2$ cup low-fat sour cream

4 halibut fillets, about 5 ounces each, skin on

1 tablespoon olive oil

Salt and pepper to taste

Garnish: sprigs of watercress

Calories 186, **Fat** (g) 7, **Carbohydrates** (g) 0, **Protein** (g) 21, **Fiber** (g) 0, **Saturated Fat** (g) 3, **Cholesterol** (mg) 46, **Sodium** (mg) 199, **ADA Exchange** 3 very lean meat

Broiled Halibut with Watercress

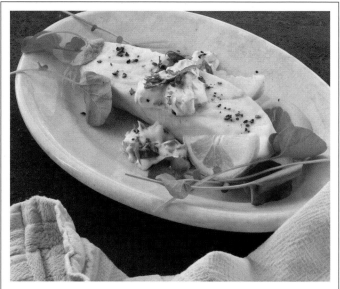

- Mix the first three ingredients together; set sauce aside. Turn on broiler; place rack about 5 inches from the heat source.

- Prepare a baking sheet with nonstick spray. Place fish, skin side down, on sheet. Drizzle with olive oil; sprinkle with salt, pepper.

- Broil fish until it starts to brown and flakes. If very thick, switch the oven to "bake" at 350°F until the fish flakes, and let it cook through.

- Serve fish with sauce on the side or drizzled on top. Garnish with sprigs of fresh watercress.

Broil a thick fillet of fish: A good firm fish like halibut can be grilled over charcoal or on a gas grill—it won't fall apart. The easiest way to cook it is to run the fish under the broiler. If it is a very thick cut, you will have to turn your oven to "bake" to cook it through. Cod and perch are preferred for deep-frying, as in fish and chips. However, a boneless fillet of halibut is fine for frying in a light batter. Dried dill weed, lemon juice, and low-fat sour cream make a delicious sauce for fish. Simply combine 1 teaspoon dried dill weed with ½ cup sour cream and 1 tablespoon freshly squeezed lemon juice.

Checking Your Fillet for Bones

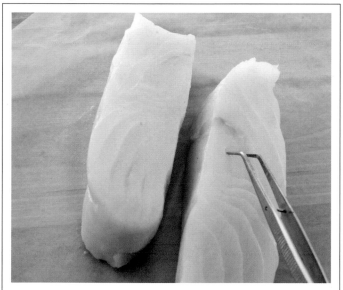

- Fish fillets are boneless; any bones found are a mistake by the fishmonger. Fish steaks have bones in them.

- Fortunately it doesn't happen often, but sometimes a bone can sneak into a fish fillet.

- You can find any bones by running your finger over the fillet, back and forth, against the grain.

- Should you find a bone, pull it out with tweezers.

- It never hurts to be extra careful.

Fillets vs. Steaks

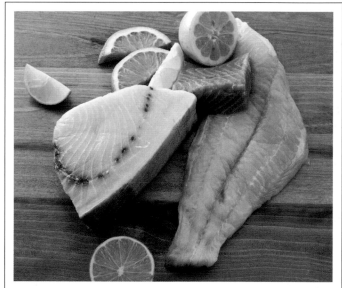

- Salmon now comes in a rolled-up steak, called a medallion. It's round and held together with either plastic webbing or its own skin.

- Large, ocean-going fish are usually marketed and served as fillets. These include black, striped, and sea bass.

- Fillets tend to be thicker at the end near the head than at the tail end. So move your broiler pan around to ensure even cooking.

CORNMEAL-CRUSTED BAKED CATFISH

If you love the crispy crust on fried fish but not the fat calories, try this recipe

There are so many ways to crust a fish; this is a very good method that is sure to please the family.

Catfish is farmraised and sold as boneless, skinless fillets that are easy to cook. You can add some Cajun spice to the fillets if your family wants a true Southern touch. Or you can simply rub them with Asian spice mix, which will give you a completely different taste experience.

Generally, it's better to make your own coating. Store-bought coating mixes are loaded with salt and/or sugar, which we can all do without. *Yield: 4 servings*

Ingredients

1 whole egg

1 egg white

¹/₂ cup cornmeal

¹/₂ cup all-purpose flour

1 teaspoon baking powder

1 teaspoon salt

1 teaspoon sweet paprika

¹/₂ teaspoon thyme

¹/₂ teaspoon garlic powder

¹/₂ teaspoon ground cumin

1 teaspoon cayenne pepper, or to taste

1 teaspoon freshly ground black pepper, or to taste

4 catfish fillets, about 5-6 ounces each

2 tablespoons olive oil, sprayed

Garnish: 4 lemon wedges and fresh parsley

Calories 256, **Fat** (g) 8, **Carbohydrates** (g) 21, **Protein** (g) 21, **Fiber** (g) 2, **Saturated Fat** (g) 2, **Cholesterol** (mg) 78, **Sodium** (mg) 774, **Carb Choices** 1½, **ADA Exchange** 1½ starch, 3 very lean meat

Cornmeal-Crusted Baked Catfish

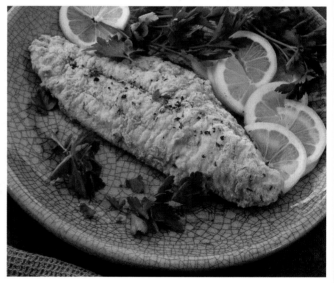

- Preheat oven to 350°F. Whisk eggs in a shallow bowl; set aside. Mix all the dry ingredients on a large piece of waxed paper.

- Dip catfish in the eggs and then roll fillets in cornmeal mixture. Press dry ingredients into the flesh, and make sure they stick.

- Arrange fillets on a baking dish prepared with nonstick spray. Lightly spray olive oil on the catfish.

- Bake 25 to 30 minutes until golden brown and crisp. Garnish with lemon wedges and parsley. Serve with your favorite sauce.

About catfish: Catfish is a sweet and delicious freshwater fish. Its natural habitat is muddy river, stream, pond, or lake—it loves mud. However, through aqua-farming, catfish are now born and raised in clean water. Farm-raised catfish have no muddy taste. Traditionally, catfish is dipped in an egg batter and then a mixture of flour and cornmeal that's been seasoned. It's then fried in deep fat. Years ago, people used lard to fry their fish; over time, a new consciousness has arisen, that of keeping food fat-free for hearrt health. As a result, this recipe calls for baking the fish in order to reduce the fat intake, but the results are no less delectable.

Checking Fish for Freshness

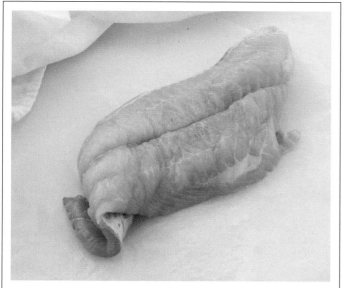

- When you buy catfish, look for a creamy color and a firm texture.

- Always smell fish before you buy it.

- Any decent fish store or supermarket fish department should be happy to put the fish on a piece of paper and let you give it a good sniff. It should smell fresh, even milky, or like the sea on a clear morning.

- When you get fish home, check freshness; make sure the flesh springs back when pressed with a fingertip. Smell it, too. If it doesn't pass the tests, take it back.

Using Citrus Zest with Fish

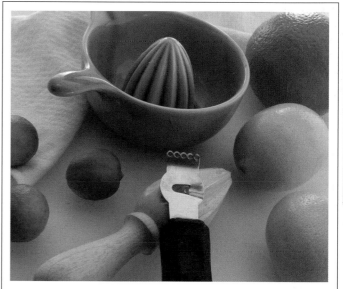

- Try using orange or lemon zest in your next breading for baked fish.

- Lime zest can get very bitter when cooked, so use it only for fresh dishes. Lime juice, however, cooks very well and maintains a tart taste without bitterness.

- A mixture of orange and lemon zest is great when added to bread crumbs for fish coatings.

- Grapefruit zest is less common; however, it can be quite good on a fish that will stand up to strong flavors.

CASHEW-CRUSTED SALMON FILLETS

The baked avocado with lime dressing in this recipe adds great flavor contrast

Using nuts with fish is a fairly new idea but one worth exploring. You will find that as the nuts brown on the fish, they develop a buttery flavor that is absolutely delicious. In this dish, it doesn't compete with the salmon at all but does make it even sweeter.

The contrast with baked avocado and lime juice is stunningly good. Try using other juices, such as tropical sour orange juice or grapefruit juice, as a substitute for the lime juice in your dressing. Other nuts, such as pine nuts, can also be used as a crust on salmon. Macadamia nuts add as many calories as a pork chop to the meal, so try to avoid them. To cut back on the fat, eliminate either oil or avocado. *Yield: 4 servings*

Ingredients

Juice of 1 lime

3 tablespoons olive oil

1/4 teaspoon salt or salt substitute

1/4 teaspoon Splenda

Tabasco sauce, a few drops or to taste

1 avocado, cut in half and pitted

4 salmon fillets, about 6 ounces each

1/3 cup whole cashews, ground coarsely in the food processor

Garnish: 4 to 8 lime wedges

Calories 538, **Fat** (g) 39, **Carbohydrates** (g) 13, **Protein** (g) 34, **Fiber** (g) 7, **Saturated Fat** (g) 8, **Cholesterol** (mg) 87, **Sodium** (mg) 241, **Carb Choice** 1, **ADA Exchange** 1 starch, 4 medium-fat meat, 3½ fat

Cashew-Crusted Salmon Fillets

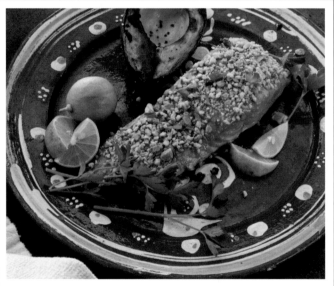

- Preheat oven to 350°F. Using a fork, whisk lime juice, oil, salt, Splenda, and Tabasco sauce in a cup. Spread mixture on avocado halves and fillets.

- Spread the ground nuts evenly on the fish fillets and press into the flesh.

- Arrange avocado halves and fish, skin side down, on a baking pan prepared with nonstick spray.

- Bake for 20 minutes, or until avocado is softened, nuts are brown, and fish is done. Serve with lime wedges on the side.

Kid-friendly ideas: Children can be fussy eaters. To appeal to them, try substituting peanuts for cashews. In any case, be sure that the nuts are raw and not preroasted, or they will get too brown and lose their delicate taste. You may well find that children who won't eat fish will try it when it looks more like a chicken tender or their favorite nut bar.

Give your kids a great reason for eating fish. Make them salmon fillets, ¼ pound per child, with fun toppings, such as 1 tablespoon of chopped tomato; a couple of olives, chopped; or chopped pieces of a peeled orange.

Grinding Nuts

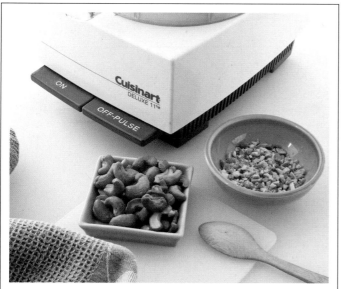

- To coarsely grind nuts, pulse them in a food processor, pausing to scrape down the sides of the bowl.

- Or grind nuts coarsely by placing them on waxed paper, covering them with another piece of waxed paper, and pounding them with a heavy cast-iron frying pan or meat mallet.

- For finely ground nuts, pulse in a food processor for a few seconds, then whirl the nuts on high.

- Don't use a blender. You will end up with unground nuts on the top and a paste at the bottom.

Flavoring Ground Nuts

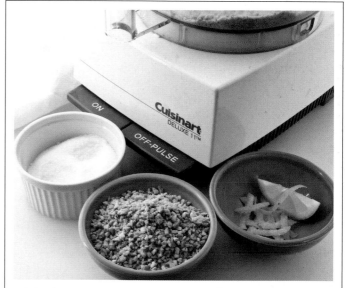

- Whether you're preparing fish, chicken breasts, or pork cutlets, nuts make a great crust.

- Always buy raw, unsalted, unroasted nuts. Then, you can add seasonings to the nutty crust that will not interfere with your recipes.

- While grinding and seasoning nuts, control your salt and sugar intake by using salt substitute and Splenda.

- Try adding dried herbs, such as thyme or rosemary. Add some lemon, orange, or grapefruit zest to nuts while you are grinding them.

SPICY BARBECUED SHARK SKEWERS

Charcoal-grilled shark is delightful when marinated or dressed in chili-citrus sauce

Shark is tender, sweet, and versatile. The only thing that will ruin a piece of shark is overcooking.

Shark is a lot like firm-fleshed swordfish, but a bit softer and milder. Making a marinade of chili sauce, orange juice, and Worcestershire sauce will enhance the fish. Grilling some orange slices along with the shark is sublime.

If you are using skewers, be sure to marinate the fish so that it has time to absorb the flavors. A slight charring is fine, but do not burn shark or any other fish.

Add orange sections to the shark on the skewers. Or add vegetables, such as chunks of zucchini, cherry tomatoes, or chunks of sweet red onion. *Yield: 4 servings*

Ingredients

2 tablespoons light (low-sodium) soy sauce

Juice of ¹/₂ sour orange or regular juice orange (used for analysis)

1 teaspoon brown Splenda

1 tablespoon low-sodium tomato paste

¹/₄ teaspoon ground cloves

Pinch of ground cinnamon

¹/₂ teaspoon garlic powder

Freshly ground black pepper to taste

1¹/₄ pounds fresh boneless shark steak, cut into 1¹/₂-inch cubes

8 wooden or metal skewers (if wood, presoak for at least 30 minutes)

Calories 185, **Fat** (g) 3, **Carbohydrates** (g) 7, **Protein** (g) 31, **Fiber** (g) 1, **Saturated Fat** (g) 1, **Cholesterol** (mg) 46, **Sodium** (mg) 292, **ADA Exchange** 1 vegetable, 4 very lean meat

Spicy Barbecued Shark Skewers

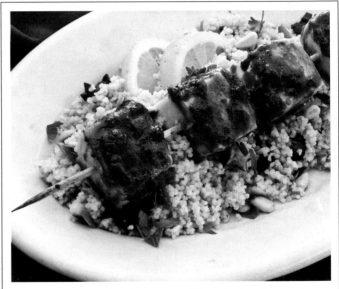

- In a large mixing bowl, whisk the first eight ingredients together.

- Add shark cubes, turning to coat. Cover and refrigerate for 1 to 2 hours, turning occasionally to coat evenly.

- Preheat grill or broiler to medium-high, about 375°F.

- Place shark cubes on skewers and grill until nicely brown.

- Cook about 3 minutes per side. Do not overcook or the shark will dry out. It's better to undercook than overcook.

Shark appetizers: Shark on skewers is a great hors d'oeuvre. Skewer shark pieces and coat with mango salsa or Asian dipping sauce. Allow ¼ pound per person. Cut into 1-inch cubes and string on wooden skewers. (Soak wooden skewers before using.) Use ½ mango, mixed with 1 teaspoon minced gingerroot and 1 teaspoon lime juice. Grill for 2 minutes per side.

Mediterranean shark skewers: Give your shark skewers a Mediterranean flavor with a marinade of 2 teaspoons olive oil, the juice of 1 lemon, and 1 teaspoon oregano for every pound of cubed shark meat. Marinate 30 minutes, then string on skewers and grill 2 minutes per side.

Skewers: Wooden or Metal?

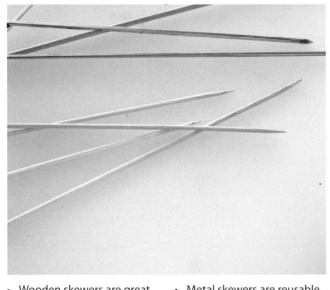

- Wooden skewers are great for grilling; however, they must be presoaked in water to prevent them from catching fire.

- Wooden skewers can be made from rosemary stems, which give food an herbal flavor. Or they can be made from cedar or ash.

- Metal skewers are reusable. They often have medallions or miniature handles on one end, which make them resemble small swords.

- Metal skewers are easily cleaned with a scouring pad. Be sure to get stainless steel if you buy metal skewers.

Shark Snacks for the Cocktail Tray

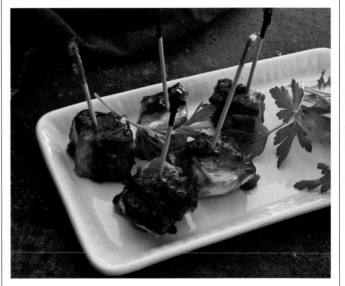

- By cutting the shark into smaller pieces, you can broil them very quickly on an attractive broiling pan, such as one in the shape of a fish.

- Prepare the pan with nonstick spray. Place the shark on the pan, then run it under a hot broiler. Turn the shark, and remove after

a few more seconds of cooking.

- Once it's cooked, spear the shark pieces with toothpicks. Let cool slightly.

- You can garnish your cocktail platter with lemon wedges.

FISH

BROILED COD OR SCROD

Codfish is one of the most versatile fish and is mostly used in fish and chips

Cod is a fine, white ocean-going fish that is popular on both sides of the Atlantic. Young cod is called scrod and is also very delicious.

Cod may be fried, as in fish and chips. It can also be baked, broiled, poached for fish chowder, or ground up as the base for codfish cakes. Codfish cakes are a staple of the frozen food department and truly delectable when homemade.

This recipe calls for broiling cod with cherry tomatoes. Cod is so low in fat that it needs some margarine or olive oil to keep it moist while cooking. Dried salt-cod is called *bacala* by the Italians and *bacalao* by the Spanish. It requires two days of soaking in fresh water and is very good. *Yield: 4 servings*

Ingredients

4 cod steaks or scrod filets (5 ounces each)

Juice of ¹/₂ lemon

16 cherry tomatoes, cut in halves

1 tablespoon fresh dill weed

Salt and pepper to taste

2 tablespoons panko breadcrumbs

a quick spray of olive oil or a drizzle of 1 tablespoon

Calories 184, **Fat** (g) 5, **Carbohydrates** (g) 8, **Protein** (g) 26, **Fiber** (g) 1, **Saturated Fat** (g) 1, **Cholesterol** (mg) 60, **Sodium** (mg) 203, **ADA Exchange** ½ starch, 3 very lean meat

Baked Cod or Scrod

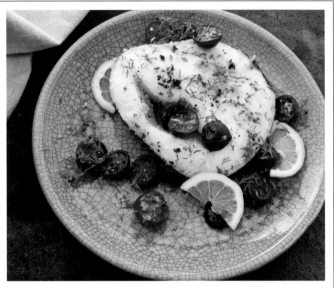

- Preheat oven to 450°F. Prepare a gratin pan or shallow casserole dish with nonstick spray.

- Arrange fish in pan. Sprinkle with lemon juice, and arrange tomato halves around fish.

- Sprinkle with dill, salt, pepper, and panko bread crumbs.

- Broil 4 to 5 minutes, or until the fish is sizzling and the bread crumbs are browned.

- Reduce heat to bake at 300°F and let finish for 3 or 4 more minutes.

Fun variations: For a wonderful variation, use mild salsa instead of fresh tomatoes. Cilantro, popular in Mexican cooking, and dill weed, a staple of Scandinavian cooking, are strong herbs worth a try. Both can be terrific with fish, but use a light touch at first.

For a crunchy crust: Another tasty variation is to coat the fish with lemon juice, spread with a thin coating of low-fat mayonnaise, and sprinkle with ¼ cup panko bread crumbs. This will give the fish a great crunchy crust and add only a few calories to the dish. Dill weed mixed with 1 part cider vinegar to 2 parts water also makes a good baking sauce for a full-bodied, rich fish.

About Panko Bread Crumbs

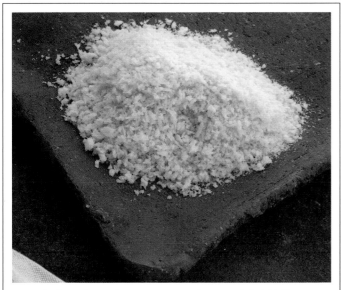

- Panko bread crumbs are popular in Southeast Asian cooking. Panko in Japanese means "bread crumbs."

- These bread crumbs are made from a light white bread somewhat like saltines or oyster crackers.

- They are delightfully crisp when used in frying and baking all kinds of meat, fish, and vegetables.

- You can buy panko bread crumbs at most supermarkets and at Asian markets.

Diabetes and Bread Crumbs

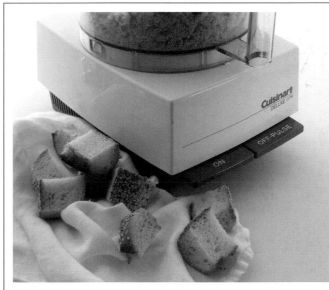

- Fresh bread crumbs are made with soft bread, which toasts nicely when used as a coating or crust.

- Toast and stale bread can also be used to make bread crumbs. Cut bread into large cubes and whirl them in a food processor.

- For flavored bread crumbs, add garlic powder, dried oregano or any other dried herb, salt, ground black or white pepper, and/or dried citrus zest.

FISH

GRANDMA'S FILLET OF SOLE

Fillet of sole is a sweet and delicate fish that's wonderful when roasted

This sautéed fillet of sole is topped with "Grandma's Crust," a combination of bread crumbs, mushrooms, and lemon zest.

The fish is served with plenty of fresh arugula. Because sole is so delicate, it's important not to overwhelm it with strong herbs, spices, or aromatic vegetables, such as garlic. If that happens, the delicate flavor is lost.

Sole (lemon, gray, or Dover) is also good served plain, broiled, and dressed simply with lemon and parsley. If you plan to roast the fish for a group, buy 5- to 6-ounce fillets per person. Ask your fishmonger how best to prepare fish for cooking. Roast the whole fish, and garnish it with lots of goodies. *Yield: 4 servings*

Ingredients

4 5-ounce sole fillets

1 tablespoon olive oil

1 tablespoon lemon juice

1 teaspoon each fresh lemon zest and fresh orange zest

Salt and freshly ground pepper to taste

$1/2$ cup fine dry bread crumbs

Garnish: sprigs of fresh parsley

Grandma's Fillet of Sole

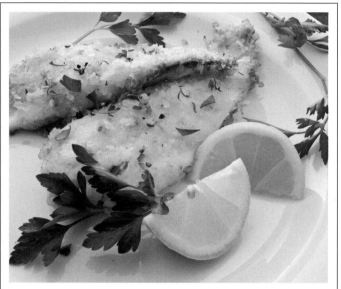

- Set sole fillets on a piece of waxed paper.

- Heat oil in a large nonstick pan over medium heat. Add olive oil. Sprinkle fish with lemon juice.

- Mix the zest, salt, pepper, and bread crumbs together. Spread on the sole.

- Sauté the sole for 3 to 4 minutes per side, until golden brown but not falling apart.

Calories 188, **Fat** (g) 5, **Carbohydrates** (g) 10, **Protein** (g) 26, **Fiber** (g) 1, **Saturated Fat** (g) 2, **Cholesterol** (mg) 59, **Sodium** (mg) 368, **ADA Exchange** 1 starch, 3 very lean meat

Light fare for people with diabetes: It's wonderful to fill up on a dish that's both satisfying and good for you. Yes, there are fat and calories in sole, but they are the "good" fats that provide healthy calories. The secret to eating when on a diet is moderation. Gobbling and gorging food just packs on calories. Taking small bites and chewing slowly will satisfy you much more completely than swallowing down gulps of food. Don't dot fish with butter before broiling or grilling. It may be delicious, but it's not a good dietary choice.

When Is the Fish Done?

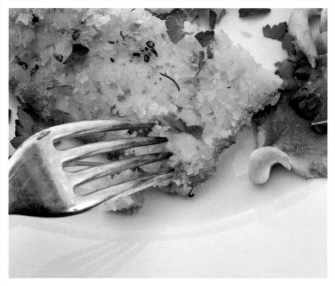

- Cookbooks used to say that fish is done when it flakes when separated with a fork.

- Today, chefs and cooks prefer not to overcook fish. Overcooking dries it out and can even make it tough.

- This method of cooking fish quickly at high heat is a good one. If the fish is very thick, you will want to brown it under the broiler and then bake it.

- Learn to listen to the fish and what to look for; listen for the sizzle, and look for a delicate browning on top. Your fish will be perfectly done.

Baking and Broiling Fish

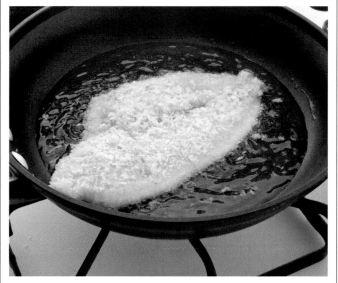

- When sautéing fish, you can make a sauce with fresh tomatoes, mushrooms, spinach, or almost anything you enjoy.

- When the fish has been turned, let cook for another 2 minutes, place on a pre-warmed plate, and cover.

- Add 4 ounces fresh spinach, or one cup fresh, chopped onions to the pan.

- If necessary, stir in 1 ounce dry white wine or 1 teaspoon extra olive oil. Keep stirring, and then add to the fish.

MUSSELS IN WHITE WINE SAUCE

Low in calories and cholesterol, mussels are an easy-to-make delicacy

This dish is a snap to prepare and a true classic. It makes a wonderful sauce that is excellent when sopped up with crusty toasted chunks of multigrain bread or served with pasta.

Mussels are a terrific source of protein. Most mussels in the market are farm raised and do not need scrubbing; but sometimes they do have "beards," which are easy to pull off.

The beards help the mussels to cling to rocks or stakes. Mussels grow well along rocky shores and in bays, inlets, and areas where the water is clean and frequently changing.

Mussels are very low in calories and very low in fat. *Yield: 4 servings*

Ingredients

3 pounds fresh live mussels

2 tablespoons olive oil

2–3 cloves garlic, peeled and chopped

1 shallot, peeled and chopped

$1/2$ bunch fresh Italian flat-leaf parsley, washed and chopped

Freshly ground black pepper to taste

$2/3$ cup dry white wine

Calories 251, **Fat** (g) 13, **Carbohydrates** (g) 4, **Protein** (g) 31, **Fiber** (g) 0, **Saturated Fat** (g) 2, **Cholesterol** (mg) 83, **Sodium** (mg) 734, **ADA Exchange** 3 medium-fat meat

Mussels in White Wine Sauce

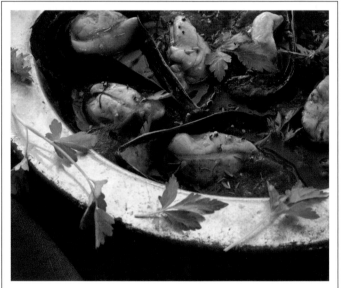

- Check mussels for cleanliness and liveliness. Rinse in cold water and remove any beards. Set aside.

- Warm oil in a large pot over medium-high heat.

- Sauté garlic and shallot for about 4 minutes, until softened. Add remaining ingredients. Add mussels; cover pot and cook over high heat until the mussels have opened.

- As mussels open, transfer them to a large bowl. A nice touch is to remove the top shell of each. Cook down the sauce, reducing it by half, and pour over mussels.

Mussels are versatile, which makes them a great dish to serve on any occasion. They can be cooked in any marinara sauce and are wonderful with ¼ cup cream added to this recipe. They mix well with garlic, and do more than well when cooked with shallots. Herbs are also outstanding with mussels. You can't go wrong by steaming mussels and serving them with a bit of melted low-fat margarine and lemon. Or try them dipped in their own broth with a touch of lemon juice. When cooked, mussels release a lot of juice. That juice, which is correctly called liqueur, is delicious. Never add salt to mussels, as they have quite a bit of salt in their systems.

Checking for Live Mussels

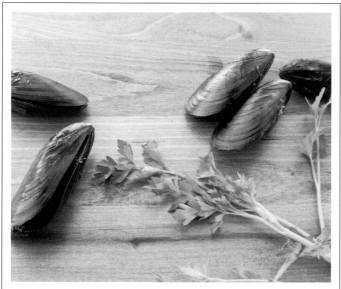

Safe Seafood

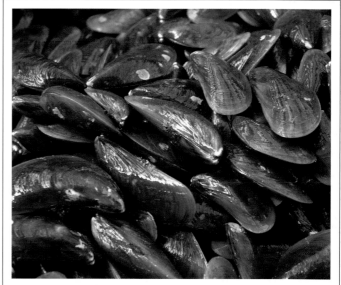

- Never, ever, cook a dead mussel. Live mussels open and close on their own. If you tap an open mussel against a closed one, it should close.

- Listen for a sharp click, not a hollow sound, when tapping mussels together. Give them all a chance to open.

- Discard any mussel that is cracked.

- Discard any mussel that does not close.

- By law, shipments of fresh raw fish and other seafood must be tagged to show area of origin—in the case of mussels, where they were harvested.

- Any reputable seafood seller should be happy to show you the area of origin. If not, go elsewhere.

- If you live on either coast, you can probably bypass the retailers and go straight to the source.

- Find out the date of collection. And remember, if a mussel doesn't close prior to cooking or doesn't open when cooked, discard it. Be safe.

SCALLOPS & SHRIMP SCAMPI

This recipe calls for baking the scallops and shrimp rather than sautéing them

This recipe can be finished at the last minute with a little leeway. Most scampi dishes are sautéed over very high heat. This one is baked, which gives you a little more time between cooking and serving.

Scallops and shrimp together are a natural combination, although scallops are mollusks and shrimp are crustaceans.

Uncooked, frozen shrimp are fine, but if you can get fresh-caught shrimp from the Gulf of Mexico, the dish will sparkle.

Bay scallops are farm raised and are cheaper than diver scallops or those from Nantucket or the tip of Long Island. The prices for shellfish vary depending on the time of year, over-fishing, and other economic variables. *Yield: 4 servings*

Ingredients

1 1/2 cups fresh bread crumbs

3 cloves garlic, peeled and chopped

1 1/2 teaspoons dried oregano

2 teaspoons sweet Hungarian paprika

Salt and freshly ground pepper to taste

1/4 cup olive oil

Juice and zest of 1/2 lemon

1/2 pound raw shrimp, peeled and cleaned

1 pound bay scallops, rinsed

Garnish: sprigs of Italian parsley and lemon wedges

Calories 451, **Fat** (g) 18, **Carbohydrates** (g) 34, **Protein** (g)34, **Fiber** (g) 3, **Saturated Fat** (g) 3, **Cholesterol** (mg) 131, **Sodium** (mg) 566, **ADA Exchange** 2 starch, 4 medium-fat meat

Scallops & Shrimp Scampi

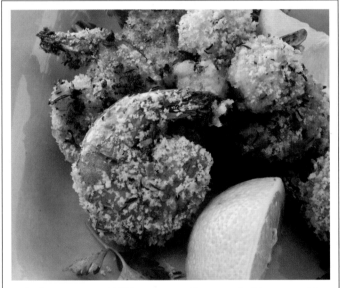

- Preheat oven to 400°F.

- Mix the first seven ingredients together, in the order listed, in a bowl large enough to hold the shrimp and scallops. Toss the seafood into the mixture and coat well.

- Prepare a baking pan with nonstick spray. Turn seafood onto the baking pan.

- Bake until the crumbs are lightly browned and the shrimp is pink. Sprinkle with sprigs of fresh parsley, and serve with fresh lemon wedges.

The fresher, the better: As long as you use fresh or frozen raw seafood, not precooked, you'll get great results in your scampi. If the seafood is precooked and you then cook it some more, it will become rubbery. If you decide to use clams, allow six cherrystones or eight littleneck clams per person. Simply open them and add them, raw, to the sauce described in this recipe.

Fun variations: Use ¼ cup grapefruit juice instead of lemon juice. Or, substitute tomato juice for its lower acid content. Add 1 cup fresh chopped tomatoes. Use ¼ pound per person of shelled king crab, stone crab, or Dungeness crabmeat. Or use uncooked lobster claws and shrimp. Add 1 ounce per person if you have to peel shrimp. Lobster meat should be parboiled.

Rinse and Dry Seafood

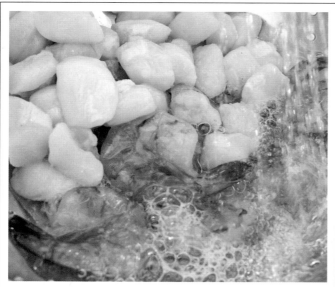

Moistening Food with Oil or Wine

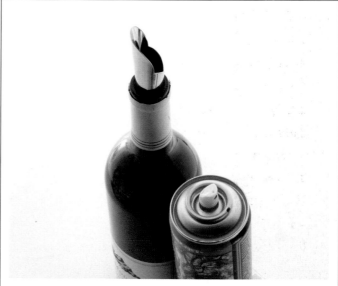

- The reason for rinsing seafood is to remove any sticky matter before cooking.

- After rinsing, dry the seafood on paper towels.

- It is important to dry the seafood if you will be baking it with crumbs so that the crumbs won't get soggy when coating the seafood.

- If you are sautéing, the water will cause your oil to snap and hiss, making it difficult to cook the seafood properly.

- Because bread crumbs vary greatly, you may need to moisten yours while baking.

- Shrimp and scallops also vary in their moisture content.

- Spraying on some extra oil or wine slows the cooking process.

SEARED DIVER SCALLOPS

Diver scallops are huge and rather expensive but definitely worth it

The sauce that accompanies these scallops has solid Carribean influences. Although the sauce itself is not strongly flavored, it is distinctive.

The sweetness of the sauce comes from the natural flavor of coconut milk. The spikiness of lime juice, hot pepper, and ginger combine for a piquant touch.

For several years, scallops were overcollected and endangered; there was a ban on the collecting and selling of these creatures. Fortunately, the ban has since been lifted. The large shells of scallops are also marketed as cooking vessels. They last for a long time and can be cleaned easily if you prepare them with cooking spray. Try it over couscous or brown rice. Balance your carbs and proteins, however, if you use them. *Yield: 4 servings*

Ingredients

For the sauce:

1 cup unsweetened coconut milk

1 teaspoon freshly ground ginger

1 teaspoon cayenne pepper, or to taste

1 teaspoon sweet Hungarian paprika

1 teaspoon Asian sesame seed oil

Juice of 1 fresh lime

Salt to taste

For the scallops:

2 tablespoons cooking oil, such as canola

1 pound diver scallops, rinsed and dried

Optional: Serve over ½ cup cooked couscous or rice per person

Garnish: sprigs of cilantro and lime wedges

Calories 288, **Fat** (g) 21, **Carbohydrates** (g) 7, **Protein** (g) 20, **Fiber** (g) 0, **Saturated Fat** (g) 12, **Cholesterol** (mg) 37, **Sodium** (mg) 191, **Carb Choice** ½, **ADA Exchange** ½ starch, 3 medium-fat meat, 1 fat

Seared Diver Scallops

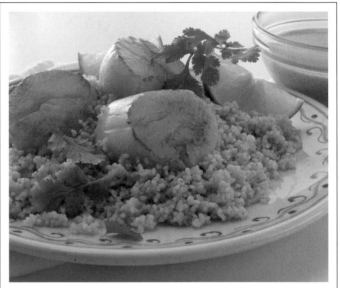

- In a saucepan, whisk all the sauce ingredients together and warm over very low heat. Set aside; keep in warm pan.

- Prepare couscous or rice, if using. Warm your plates.

- Heat cooking oil in a nonstick pan over high heat. Add scallops, and sear quickly until golden brown on each side, no more than 1 minute per side.

- Arrange scallops over couscous or rice, if using. Spoon sauce over the top of each serving and garnish.

All about scallops: Scallops come in small (bay scallops), medium, large, and jumbo (diver) sizes. Diver scallops can weigh up to 2 ounces each. They are sweet and succulent, and only get tough if overcooked. Don't worry about cooking them through—you just want them to be hot inside and seared on the outside.

With a cajun accent: Affordable bay scallops can be used in spicy Cajun dishes. Coat 1 pound scallops with a sprinkling of paprika, white pepper, and allspice, then fry the scallops in 2 teaspoons olive oil for 2 to 3 minutes. Your favorite light cream sauce will help keep the heat under control. Serve over brown rice with a medley of vegetables on the side.

Hot Food and Cold Plates Don't Mix

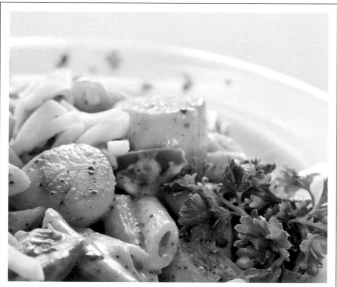

- A well-trained chef will warm plates for hot food and chill plates for cold food.

- Newer ovens have a separate warming area. Or, you can just put the plates over an asbestos or flameproof grid on the stovetop on the lowest possible setting.

- Hot trays are excellent for buffets when you wish to keep both the food and the plates warm.

- When serving cold entree salads or desserts, simply put the plates in the refrigerator for a while, especially on a hot day.

Garnishes for Caribbean-Style Dishes

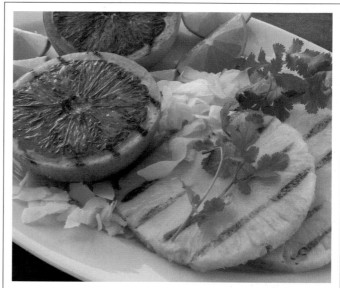

- Aside from limes and cilantro, there are many fun things to use as garnishes for these exotic dishes.

- Small chunks of grilled pineapple, shredded fresh coconut, and broiled coconut chips are all wonderful.

- Try serving a grilled grapefruit half on the side of each portion. Avocados, sliced and sprinkled with lime juice, are also very colorful and tasty.

- Note that these garnishes are not in the analysis of this dish, and they add carbs and fat.

BAKED STUFFED CHERRYSTONES

A New England favorite, these clams are lower in fat and calories than most

Every cook and chef who loves baked stuffed clams has his or her own special recipe, which is often kept as a family or restaurant secret. But now we're unleashing this secret recipe, which is guaranteed to become a family favorite.

Cherrystone clams are about 2 inches in diameter, whereas chowder clams are much bigger, but even chowder clams do get tender when minced and cooked (never overcook, or you'll get rubber).

There are ways to mix up this dish with a variety of other ingredients and flavors, such as bacon, Parmesan cheese, or pancetta. But be sure to stick within the restrictions of your diet. *Yield 6 servings*

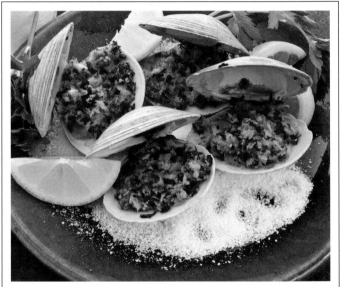

Baked Stuffed Cherrystone Clams

Ingredients

6 cherrystone clams (reserve juice)

¹/₄ cup water

2 tablespoons olive oil

¹/₂ cup shallots, peeled and minced

2 cloves garlic, peeled and minced

¹/₄ cup diced smoked ham (used in analysis) or cooked turkey bacon, crumbled

1 teaspoon dried oregano

2 tablespoons fresh Italian flat-leaf parsley, minced

¹/₂ cup grated Parmesan cheese

1 cup dry bread crumbs

Freshly ground black pepper to taste

1 tablespoon dry white wine or reserved clam cooking liquid to moisten, if necessary

Garnish: fresh lemon wedges

Calories 88, **Fat** (g) 4, **Carbohydrates** (g) 8, **Protein** (g) 5, **Fiber** (g) 1, **Saturated Fat** (g) 1, **Cholesterol** (mg) 7, **Sodium** (mg) 168, **Carb Choice** ½, **ADA Exchange** ½ starch

- Preheat oven to 375°F. Place clams in a pot with water; cover. Steam clams over high heat. When open, in 4 to 6 minutes, remove to a bowl; set aside. Strain off sand. Save juice.

- Twist shells apart; place them on a baking sheet. Remove clam meat and grind in food processor. Sauté shallots, garlic in fry pan in oil over medium heat. Add next seven ingredients and ground clams to pan. Mix.

- Prepare shells with nonstick spray. Spoon stuffing into shells. Bake 15 to 20 minutes, or until lightly brown and hot. Garnish. Serve.

Small clams: If you decide to make baked clams with the smaller littleneck clams, you will need to have your fishmonger open them for you. Insist that he or she save the juices for you. Littleneck clams are very tender and should be salty and sweet at the same time. The flavor of any clam comes from the water in which it lives. If you use littlenecks, you do not have to grind them, unlike cherrystones. Simply combine the clam liqueur with 1 minced garlic clove, 1 tablespoon olive oil, and 1 teaspoon lemon juice; mix with ½ cup bread crumbs, and spread on the six open clam halves. Bake them in a 375°F oven for 5 to 7 minutes, or until lightly browned.

Preparing Clams for Cooking

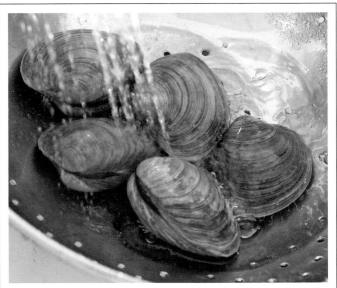

Opening Clams by Hand

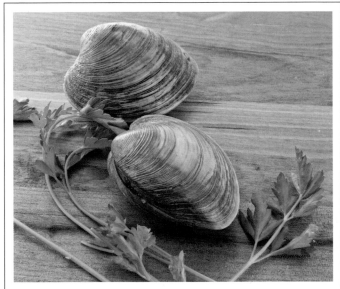

- Always scrub clams under cold running water to remove any sand.

- Discard any clams that are cracked or remain open.

- Tap all of the clams together to make sure that there is a sharp click, not a hollow thud. This ensures that the clam is alive. Never use dead clams.

- Discard any clams that do not open in the process of steaming.

- Small clams that you are not going to steam need to be opened by hand.

- Open them after they are well scrubbed and tested for liveliness.

- Hold a clam in a kitchen towel. Insert the blade of a clam knife into the crack.

- This takes skill, but will go quickly after some practice.

- When the knife is between the two halves, twist it. Working over a bowl to catch the liquid, remove the top shell and loosen the clam by running your knife around the bottom shell.

SHELLFISH

SAUTÉED SOFT-SHELL CRABS

Available from late April through June, soft-shell crabs are a springtime delicacy

Soft-shell crabs are increasingly difficult to get because of worldwide pollution. In addition, many are exported to Asian countries, where they are a delicacy, commanding huge prices.

Soft-shell crabs are a treat that can only be had at certain times of the year because of their seasonality. While they're not available year-round, they are well worth the wait.

Sautéed soft-shell crabs require just the tiniest bit of flour, not a lot of breading. Olive oil mixed with canola or peanut oil is the cooking medium of choice, not butter.

You can buy soft shell-crabs live, but then you have to clean them. It's easier to buy them precleaned. *Yield: 4 servings*

Ingredients

8 large (3 to 4 inches across) or 12 small (3 inches across) soft-shell crabs

Juice of ¹/₂ fresh lemon

Salt and cayenne pepper to taste

Quick-mixing flour (Wondra)

¹/₄ cup mixture of olive and canola oil

¹/₂ cup slivered raw almonds

Garnish: lemon halves

Calories 368, **Fat** (g) 22, **Carbohydrates** (g) 10, **Protein** (g) 32, **Fiber** (g) 2, **Saturated Fat** (g) 3, **Cholesterol** (mg) 97, **Sodium** (mg) 560, **Carb Choice** ½, **ADA Exchange** ½ starch, 4 very lean meat

Sautéed Soft-Shell Crabs

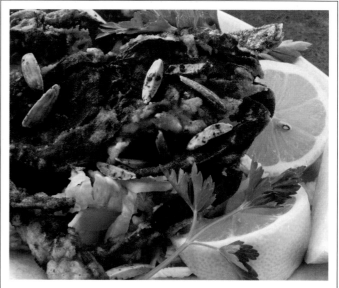

- Rinse crabs in cold water and dry with paper towels. Sprinkle with lemon juice.

- Sprinkle crabs on both sides with salt and cayenne pepper; dust with flour.

- In a large frying pan, heat oil to the smoking stage.

Add crabs and brown quickly on both sides. Drain crabs on paper towels.

- In the same pan, sauté almonds until lightly golden. Place crabs on warm plates and sprinkle with almonds. Garnish with lemon wedges.

More about crabs: Crabs range in size from 1 to 4 inches in diameter. Their shells should be tender and edible. Like any seafood, make sure the crabs smell fresh. The soft shell comes about after the hard shell is sloughed off and before a new, larger one is formed. Once the new, hard shell is on the crab, the crab's flavor and your cooking technique are affected. Crab shacks serve hard-shell crabs on picnic tables covered with newspapers. Mallets for cracking and pots of drawn butter come with the crabs, which are steamed in a giant vat. The challenge is in picking every morsel out of the claws and body of each and every crab.

A Soft-Shell Crab Sauce

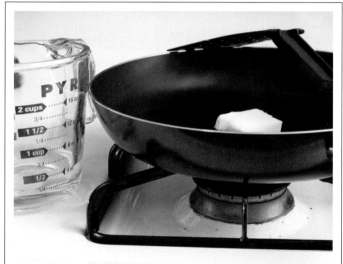

- This sauce will add a bit of flavor and interest to your crabs.

- While the crabs are draining, move the sautéed almonds to a bowl. Stir ½ cup dry white wine, such as Chardonnay, into the pan.

- Bring to a boil. Add a pat of sweet butter to the pan.

- Return the nuts to the sauté pan, and pour over the crabs.

Tartar Sauce for Crabs

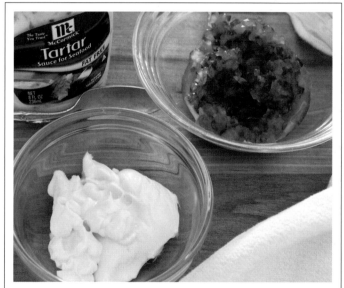

- Tartar sauce is the perfect accompaniment to most fish and other seafood.

- Bottled tartar sauce contains a lot of sugar and salt. It is easy to make your own healthier version.

- Simply mix 1 tablespoon sweet green relish (hot dog relish) with ½ cup low-fat mayonnaise.

- Mix in 2 tablespoons lemon juice and a dash of cayenne pepper, and your sauce is ready.

MIXED SEAFOOD BROIL

Say hello to spring or farewell to summer with this seafood feast

This recipe is especially great to serve when you are opening up your patio for spring or closing it in the fall.

You can make a series of dipping sauces for your mixed seafood platter. Change it up by occasion, mood, or even the weather. Cooking seafood on a metal platter or baking pan on the grill adds a wonderful smoky flavor that is enhanced with mesquite chips.

Plan on using ½ pound of shellfish per person. Remember, shells are heavy.

To cut back on the calories, try eating the seafood with just a bit of lemon juice or an olive oil and garlic mixture. *Yield: 8 servings*

Ingredients

For the basting sauce:

1 cup homemade chili sauce, sugar-free or low-sugar

Juice of ¹/₂ lemon

2 strips orange peel

¹/₄ cup cooking oil

For the seafood:

24 littleneck clams, cleaned and checked for liveliness (see page 000)

24 mussels, cleaned and checked for liveliness (see page 163)

2 live lobsters, cut into sections. Remove claws, knuckles, and cut tails in 2-inch chunks crosswise; or 2 pounds Alaskan crabs, cut into 2-inch chunks; or 2 pounds Alaska king crab legs, cut into 2-inch chunks

1 pound jumbo or colossal shrimp, with shells

Calories 276, **Fat** (g) 9, **Carbohydrates** (g) 7, **Protein** (g) 43, **Fiber** (g) 1, **Saturated Fat** (g) 1, **Cholesterol** (mg) 165, **Sodium** (mg) 1295, **Carb Choice** ½, **ADA Exchange** ½ starch, 1 lean meat

Mixed Seafood Broil

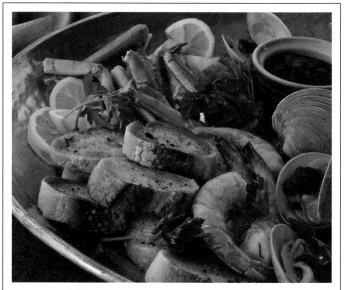

- Heat broiler or set grill on high. Mix sauce ingredients in a bowl. Wash all of the seafood and pat dry.

- Place seafood on a metal pan to be cooked in stages in the order listed at left.

- Start broiling or grilling clams and mussels; when they start to open, add lobster or crab, and, if using live lobster, cook until it turns red. When everything is almost done, add shrimp. Cook until shrimp turn pink.

- As seafood opens, brush with sauce. Let guests peel their own shrimp.

This recipe calls for a variety of seafood, cooked in stages. You put the shrimp on last, as it cooks faster than the rest. You can use any local crabmeat: blue, brown, stone crab, or Dungeness crab legs. Crab species vary by area. Blue crabs are indigenous to the East Coast; stone crabs to Florida and the Gulf of Mexico. The Dungeness crab is a specialty from the Northwest, and the king crab belongs to Alaska. When lobsters are plentiful and not overly expensive, they make an excellent addition to this mixed platter. Unshelled shrimp, the bigger the better, are fine. Clams and mussels in their shells will pop open when the heat hits them.

Cooking with Scallops and Shrimp

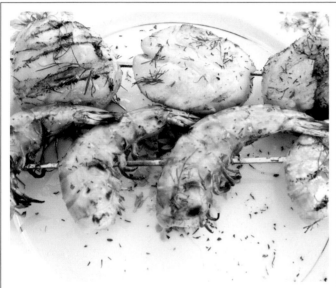

Saucing Your Seafood

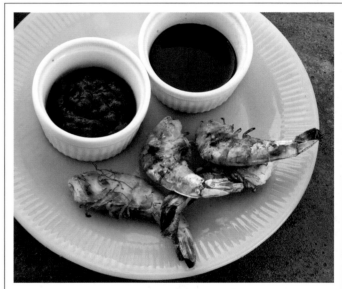

- Always put shrimp and scallops on the grill or in the broiler last.

- They will cook up fast; shrimp often will only need about 30 seconds per side. Uncooked shrimp will turn light pink in color and coil into the shape of a C.

- Start grilling or broiling clams, then add mussels or lobster chunks.

- If you are using precooked and frozen king crab, defrost it and put it on with the shrimp and scallops.

- Adding sauce to seafood while on the grill or in the broiler seals in the natural flavors.

- After you've grilled the seafood, offer your guests an Asian dipping sauce that starts with ½ cup soy sauce. Add 1 teaspoon each of minced fresh gingerroot, lemon juice, and sesame oil.

- Classic cocktail sauce is always very good. Just mix ½ cup chili sauce with 1 teaspoon each of Worcestershire, horseradish, and lemon juice.

- Any simple vinaigrette also is terrific with seafood.

BASIC POLENTA

As an appetizer or side dish, polenta is so simple, so versatile, so delicious

Polenta is cooked cornmeal, a staple of the Native American diet and a key ingredient in Italian cooking. It can be served soft and warm, or allowed to harden for grilling and sautéing. It's a high-fiber food that can be reheated and used again the next day. Liven up basic polenta with the addition of various ingredients. It is especially tasty when topped with tomato sauce, meat gravies, seafood, or grilled vegetables.

Premade polenta is a bit expensive. Because it's so very simple to make, it's not necessary to buy it. If you make two recipes at once, you can turn half of it into a polenta roll and refrigerate it for a few days or freeze it for up to a month. *Yield: 8 servings*

Ingredients

4 cups water

1 teaspoon salt

1 cup coarse-ground cornmeal

Freshly ground black pepper to taste

Optional:

¼ cup grated Parmesan cheese

½ bunch parsley, rinsed and chopped

1 tablespoon dried rosemary, or 3 tablespoons fresh, chopped

Calories 55, **Fat** (g) 1, **Carbohydrates** (g) 12, **Protein** (g) 43, **Fiber** (g) 1, **Saturated Fat** (g) 0, **Cholesterol** (mg) 0, **Sodium** (mg) 296, **Carb Choice** 1, **ADA Exchange** 1 starch

Basic Polenta

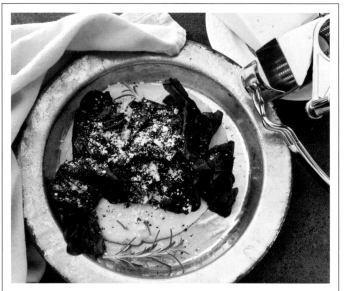

- Bring salted water to a boil in a heavy-bottomed pot (nonstick is best).

- Add cornmeal in a thin stream, very slowly. Stir it constantly with a wooden spoon.

- Keep stirring until polenta reaches the consistency of mashed potatoes. Add black pepper.

- If desired, add grated Parmesan cheese, herbs, or whatever you desire.

Enhanced polenta: This recipe can be made richer by substituting 4 cups 1 percent milk for water and adding 1 tablespoon low-fat margarine. Add ½ cup grated Parmesan cheese when the polenta is almost ready to serve. The cheese melts into the hot polenta for a savory flavor. Or, add 2 tablespoons extra-virgin olive oil to the hot polenta for a smooth consistency.

Adding herbs: Various herbs, fresh and dried, make excellent variations. A generous pinch or two of basil, marjoram, oregano, and rosemary is recommended. You can use herbs individually or in combination. A quarter cup of chopped fresh parsley is also a terrific addition. Remember, dried herbs are far more concentrated than fresh, so use less and taste often.

Stir Polenta Constantly

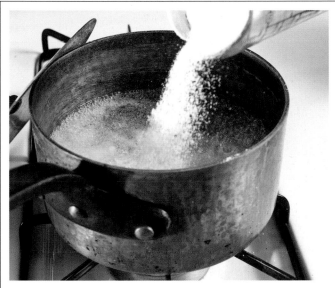

- There is a good reason for adding the cornmeal slowly and stirring it constantly.

- If you add the cornmeal all at once, you will end up with a gummy clump that cannot be saved.

- What you want is smooth, creamy polenta. Going slow and stirring constantly will result in a lovely, smooth texture.

- For a thicker consistency, increase the cooking time by a minute or two.

Making Polenta More Healthful

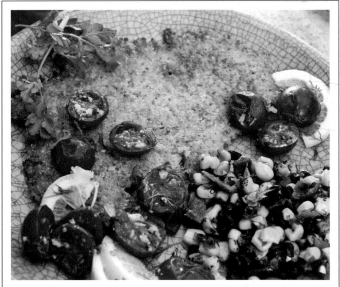

- Adding vegetables to polenta will make it more attractive and healthful by adding fiber.

- One cup of grilled, chopped vegetables turns polenta into a wonderful side dish.

- Grilled and chopped cherry tomatoes are another tasty way to make your polenta healthful.

- Add the vegetables, then bake the polenta with ¼ cup Parmesan cheese sprinkled on top.

169

SAUTÉED POLENTA

Sautéed until golden brown, polenta can be fresh and fragrant or saucy and spicy

Polenta can be formed into squares or circles for sautéing. Traditionally, polenta is sautéed in butter or deep fried in oil. We do not recommend either of these methods, as they load on the calories—big time! Instead, we do recommend a skim of olive or canola oil or nonstick spray in the sauté pan.

Serve sautéed polenta dressed with onions and black beans for lunch. Or top polenta squares or circles with a hearty tomato sauce, sliced black olives, and a sprinkling of Parmesan cheese for a light supper. Polenta can be made spicy with the addition of red pepper flakes or chopped, canned chipotle peppers. Make mini cakes and load salsa or guacamole on top for a fabulous football party snack. *Yield: 4 servings*

Ingredients

1 tablespoon olive oil

$1/2$ cup onions, finely chopped

2 cloves garlic, peeled and finely chopped

1 teaspoon dried oregano or other favorite herbs

$1/4$ cup cooked corn (optional)

$1/4$ cup finely chopped hot or sweet peppers (optional)

1 recipe (about 4 cups) cooked polenta, still warm (see recipe, page 168)

1 tablespoon canola or olive oil

Sautéed Polenta

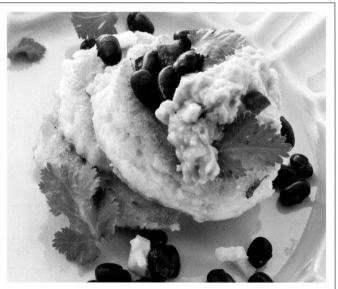

Calories 108, **Fat** (g) 5, **Carbohydrates** (g) 14, **Protein** (g) 4, **Fiber** (g) 1, **Saturated Fat** (g) 1, **Cholesterol** (mg) 4, **Sodium** (mg) 234, **Carb Choice** 1, **ADA Exchange** 1 starch, 1 fat

- Place a large, nonstick pan over medium heat. Add oil, onion, and garlic; stir. Cook until softened, about 4 minutes. Stir in oregano, corn, and peppers. Add polenta.

- Coat a sheet of heavy-duty aluminum foil with nonstick spray. Spread polenta on the foil and smooth evenly.

- Cover with plastic wrap and refrigerate for at least 2 hours.

- Cut polenta into circles.

- Heat oil in a large, nonstick skillet on medium-high. Sauté polenta cakes until golden brown on both sides.

Cooked polenta may be smoothed onto heavy-duty aluminum foil coated with nonstick spray. When hot, polenta doesn't hold its shape. As it cools, it congeals, and then you can cut it into squares or circles with a cookie cutter. Or, cook polenta the day before and spread it on foil, cover with plastic, and refrigerate overnight. Don't make squares or patties with hot polenta—they won't hold.

Flavoring polenta: While the polenta is still hot, stir in ¼ cup Parmesan cheese, 1 tablespoon of your favorite dried herbs, ¼ cup minced onions, ¼ cup cooked corn and/or chopped peppers, or whatever you plan to use as flavoring. You can give sautéed polenta cakes a Thanksgiving touch. Try this recipe instead of the usual mashed potatoes.

Sautéing Food

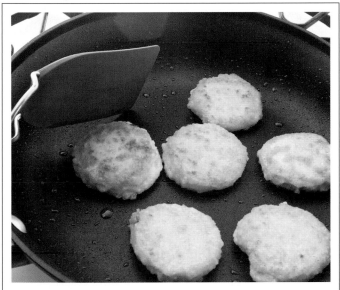

- The sauté technique is the basis of many recipes. It's a simple way to prepare highly flavorful meals.

- Sauté pans come in all sizes. Use a 7-inch pan for single-serving dishes; a 10-inch pan for double servings. Start with a tiny bit of oil over medium heat in a nonstick pan. Add food to be sautéed. Turn when either lightly browned or softened. For crisp results, preheat your pan before adding oil.

- Be sure the food is at room temperature before sautéeing.

Working with Warm Polenta

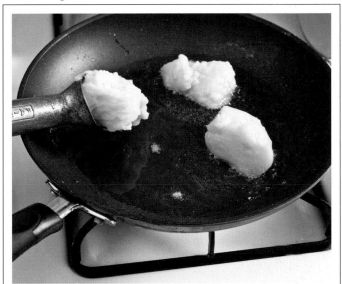

- Allow the polenta to harden, then cut into leftover soups, such as chicken or turkey.

- If you do not have time to let the polenta cool prior to sautéing it, scoop it up with an ice-cream scoop and place it in the freezer on wax paper for 10 minutes.

- If your polenta is still warm, however, it will take less time to cook.

- While it's in the pan, smooth the top down with the back of the ice-cream scoop. When it's nicely browned on one side, turn it.

QUINOA RISOTTO WITH CHICKPEAS

Quinoa is highly nutritious and works well with lots of different flavors and textures

Quinoa is grown in Bolivia, Ecuador, and Peru. It is a complete food, higher in protein than any other grain. Quinoa sustained the people of the Andes for thousands of years before the Spanish arrived. It is ideally suited for cultivation in otherwise desolate mountain areas. Thinking the quinoa "barbaric," the Spanish destroyed it, thereby reducing the natives to starvation. The crops introduced by the Spanish did not grow at high altitudes. Fortunately, quinoa is making a comeback. Cooks love its versatility: It's usable for breakfast, lunch, and dinner, as part of a main course, or as a side dish. Aside from its high-protein characteristics, quinoa is good for the digestive system—and it's delicious. *Yield: 6 servings*

Ingredients

1 cup low-salt or salt-free vegetable or chicken broth

$^1/_2$ cup water

2 tablespoons olive oil

$^1/_2$ cup finely chopped onions

1 clove garlic, peeled and chopped

1 cup quinoa, rinsed and drained

1 tablespoon dried rosemary

1 teaspoon dried oregano

1 13-ounce can chickpeas, rinsed and drained

2 tablespoons red wine vinegar

Garnish (optional): chopped tomatoes, olives, capers, freshly chopped parsley

Calories 228, **Fat** (g) 7, **Carbohydrates** (g) 35, **Protein** (g) 7, **Fiber** (g) 5, **Saturated Fat** (g) 1, **Cholesterol** (mg) 0, **Sodium** (mg) 278, **Carb Choices** 2, **ADA Exchange** 2 starch, 1 fat

Quinoa Risotto with Chickpeas

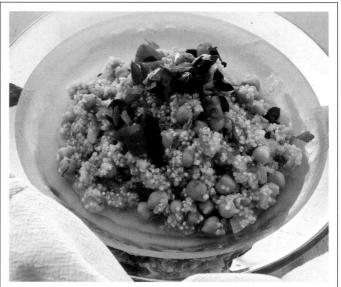

- Place broth and water in a saucepan over medium heat to warm.

- Place oil in a large pot over medium heat. Add onion, garlic, and quinoa; stir to mix.

- Slowly add warm broth/water mixture to quinoa, stirring constantly. As soon as it's absorbed and the pot begins to hiss, add a bit more. When all of the liquid is absorbed, stir in rosemary, oregano, chickpeas, and vinegar.

- Serve warm, cool, or at room temperature; garnish as desired.

Quinoa can be cooked like rice, in boiling water, or like risotto. Make quinoa risotto with pumpkin by combining 2 cups cooked pumpkin meat with 2 cups quinoa. Add leftover cooked chicken, seafood, or grilled vegetables to make a big dinner, or add 1 cup each of snow peas, baby carrots, and cherry tomatoes for a lighter entrée. Quinoa is great for people trying to add more fiber to their diets.

Finding quinoa: Although it's neither Mexican nor Spanish, quinoa is beginning to appear in the Spanish-Mexican sections of supermarkets. It is available in many health food/natural food chains and is easy to order on the Internet.

Rinse Your Quinoa and Beans

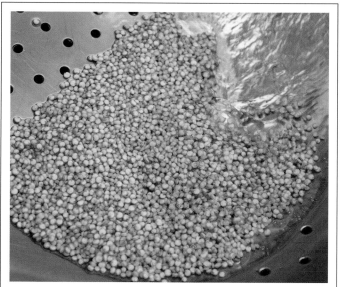

- Rinsing quinoa in a fine sieve will clean it of dirt, dust, and foreign bodies, which will appear when the quinoa is wet.

- You must also rinse dried beans such as lentils, black and pink beans, great northerns, and pintos. Like quinoa, beans often contain pebbles

and little lumps of dirt.

- A pebble can break a tooth, which is an expensive and avoidable problem.

- A lump of dirt can dissolve when liquids are added, changing the taste of the whole dish.

Slow Addition of Liquids

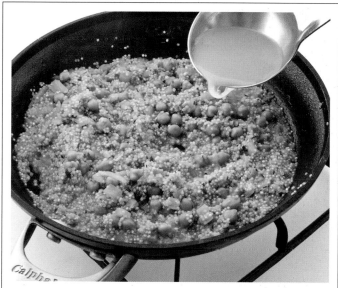

- You can boil quinoa just like rice, which sometimes results in a grainy consistency.

- The texture is much nicer if you cook it like risotto. The food will tell you when to add another half-ladle of liquid—it will make slight hissing noises.

- Don't let the onions scorch. As soon as the liquid absorbs, add another half ladle of broth.

- Watch the quinoa carefully. It takes about 20 minutes to add in all the liquid, but you'll be so happy with the results.

SEASONED BROWN RICE

More nutritious than white rice, brown rice has fiber and is very versatile

Brown rice is unprocessed, unpolished, unhulled rice. To get rice to the stage where it is white, the nutritious outer hull is removed through chemicals or a polishing process. The rice bran, the best part nutritionally, is then used to make bran muffins and bran-based cereals.

Thus, brown rice has more flavor, making it far tastier than white rice. Like white rice, brown rice lends itself to a myriad of wonderful food combinations, from the simplest recipes such as this one to the addition of meat, poultry, and seafood. Leftover rice is very useful in many next-day dishes, such as salads, soups, and stews. It stores very well in the refrigerator for up to a week. *Yield: 6 servings*

Ingredients

2 tablespoons olive oil

1 cup chopped sweet onions (such as Bermuda or Vidalia)

2 tablespoons fresh rosemary leaves or 1 tablespoon dried rosemary

1 cup brown rice

1 ³/₄ cups water, chicken broth, or vegetable broth

Pinch of salt

Freshly ground black pepper or hot pepper sauce to taste

Calories 169, **Fat** (g) 5, **Carbohydrates** (g) 27, **Protein** (g) 4, **Fiber** (g) 2, **Saturated Fat** (g) 1, **Cholesterol** (mg) 0, **Sodium** (mg) 142, **Carb Choices** 2, **ADA Exchange** 2 starch, 1 fat

Seasoned Brown Rice

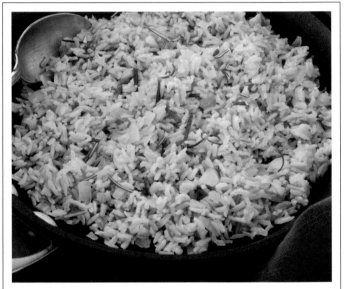

- Preheat oven to 350°F. In a large stew pot, Dutch oven, or deep frying pan, heat oil over medium heat.

- Add onions and stir, cooking about 3 minutes or until translucent. Stir in rosemary and rice, mixing to coat well. Add liquid, salt, and pepper.

- Bring to a boil. Cover and place in oven for 40 minutes.

- Remove from oven. Fluff rice and re-cover. Let stand another 10 minutes.

Quick-cooking rice with dried fruit: Following the directions on the box, prepare 4 servings (2 cups) of quick-cooking brown rice.

As soon as the rice is cooked, add 1 cup minced and sautéed onions; 1 apple, peeled, cored and chopped; ¼ cup dried cranberries; ¼ cup toasted walnuts; 1 stalk celery, rinsed and minced; 1 teaspoon dried thyme leaves; and 1 teaspoon fresh lemon zest. Stir to mix, and serve as a side dish.

Using the Proper Pots and Pans

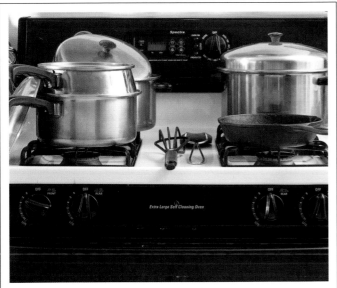

- It's best to use a heavy-bottomed, nonstick pot or Dutch oven for this recipe.

- If you use a thin metal pot, your food will stick and burn. You want slow, even heat.

- You can even use an old-fashioned, heavy-duty, 3-inch-deep cast-iron frying pan, if you have one with a lid.

- Be sure the lid you use fits tightly in order to keep the steam from escaping.

Make Extra Brown Rice

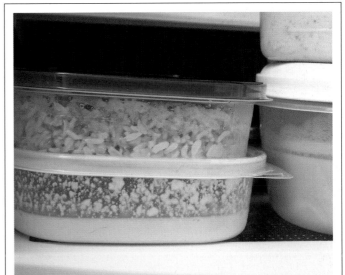

- Boil or bake a couple of extra cups of brown rice. You'll then be set for tonight's dinner, with leftovers to have for lunch as the base for a salad or as part of another dinner.

- Wise family cooks always make extra quantities of staples like brown rice, whole-wheat dough, quinoa, and polenta.

- If you want to lower your blood sugar or work on increasing your energy expenditure, it's important to plan ahead.

- Plan your food, exercise time, and some down time.

HIGH-FIBER FOODS

BROWN RICE, CHICKEN, & OLIVES

Brown rice is a great base for dishes with chicken, seafood, pork, and aromatic vegetables

This recipe is a delightful combination of harmonious flavors. It's a surprise to find how cooking changes the taste of green olives. You will detect some of the tartness from the olives, but it will meld into the rice and chicken for a subtle overall taste. Lemon and olives are also a natural combination that makes this dish special.

You can double the recipe and serve it for company. It has a slightly earthy, rustic flair, and it's also very good for people with diabetes because it's high in fiber and protein and low in fat. Plus, rice is a carb that will absorb more slowly into the bloodstream, a definite plus. *Yield: 6 servings*

Ingredients

$^1/_2$ cup olive oil

1 whole chicken, bone-in, about $2^1/_2$ pounds, cut into 6 serving pieces

2 tablespoons all-purpose flour

1 teaspoon sea salt or other light salt

$^1/_2$ teaspoon ground black pepper

1 teaspoon sweet paprika

$^1/_2$ cup coarsely chopped onions

2 cloves garlic, smashed and peeled

$1^1/_2$ cups uncooked brown rice

$1^3/_4$ cups chicken broth or a mixture of broth and wine

$^1/_2$ cup small green, pimiento-stuffed olives

1 tablespoon fresh rosemary

Juice of $^1/_2$ lemon

Calories 497, **Fat** (g) 20, **Carbohydrates** (g) 50, **Protein** (g) 29, **Fiber** (g) 3, **Saturated Fat** (g) 4, **Cholesterol** (mg) 30, **Sodium** (mg) 678, **Carb Choices** 3, **ADA Exchange** 3 starch, 3 medium-fat meat, 1 fat

Brown Rice, Chicken, & Olives

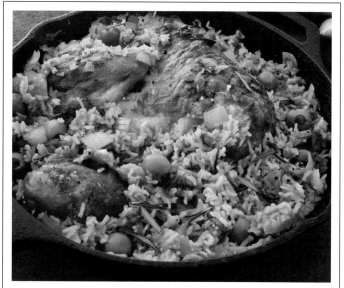

- In a large pot, heat oil over medium heat. Rinse chicken and pat dry. Mix the next four ingredients on a large piece of waxed paper. Roll chicken in the flour mixture.

- Brown chicken in oil; remove to a plate. Sauté onions and garlic in the oil until soft, about 3 minutes.

- Add rice to sautéed onions and garlic, mixing to coat well. Add liquid, and return chicken to pot. Add olives, rosemary, and lemon juice.

- Cover; bake 50 to 60 minutes at 350°F. Let rest, lid off, 5 minutes before serving.

Brown rice with Anjou pears: When cooking this dish, you may want to substitute pears for olives to make a savory/sweet dish. Stir in 2 peeled, cored, and chopped Anjou pears in place of the olives. The pears, combined with a pinch of thyme or rosemary, will change the dish completely.

Brown rice with capers: Another wonderful alternative to olives is to add 1 tablespoon capers with a pinch of oregano. If you are serving grown-ups, add 1 tablespoon green peppercorns, plus an assortment of your favorite herbs. Also for an adults-only gathering, add ½ cup dry white wine to the cooking liquid. For a very sophisticated flavor, use 1 tablespoon each of capers and dry white vermouth instead of white wine.

Brown Rice on the Stove

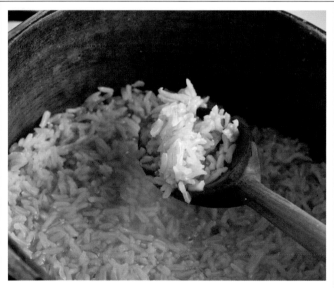

- When you boil rice on the stovetop, you have to watch it closely; it's easy to burn it or get a sticky mess on the bottom of the pan.

- Use a nonstick pan; prepare it with nonstick spray, even though you may use canola oil, olive oil, or butter in the recipe later.

- Stir often. If the rice gets dry, add more broth or water. You want the rice to be perfectly done, and brown rice is difficult to overcook.

- If you are rushed and don't want to deal with a time-consuming project, use quick-cooking brown rice.

Don't Overload Rice with Liquids

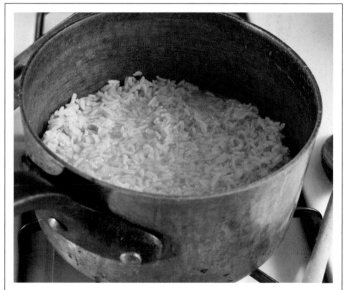

- It's better to start with package directions.

- Depending on your elevation and the humidity, cooking time will vary, as will amounts of moisture.

- Use a fork to stir the rice often, and add additional water or broth to help keep the rice from drying out.

HIGH-FIBER FOODS

WHEAT BERRIES WITH VEGETABLES
Wheat berries are a terrific source of fiber and a wonderful addition to any diet

Wheat berries work great in a slow cooker. Put 2 cups of wheat berries in a Crock-Pot in the morning with at least 1½ quarts water, but no salt. Set it on low, cover it, and go to work.

If the wheat berries aren't done when you get home, turn the Crock-Pot temperature up and add more water if necessary. Check occasionally. If they aren't done before you go to bed, turn the Crock-Pot temperature down and add more water, if necessary.

When the wheat berries are done, they will still be chewy and make a wonderful addition to soups, stews, and salads. With herbs and a salt substitute, they are excellent snacks when watching TV or munching while you work. *Yield: 6 servings*

KNACK DIABETES COOKBOOK

Ingredients

2 cups wheat berries

2 quarts water

2 tablespoons olive oil

1 cup finely chopped red onions

2 sweet red or green peppers, chopped

2 stalks celery, cleaned and chopped

1 fennel bulb, cut into thin slices

1 teaspoon orange zest

Salt and pepper to taste

Calories 175, **Fat** (g) 5, **Carbohydrates** (g) 27, **Protein** (g) 5, **Fiber** (g) 5, **Saturated Fat** (g) 1, **Cholesterol** (mg) 0, **Sodium** (mg) 451, **ADA Exchange** 2 starch

Wheat Berries with Vegetables

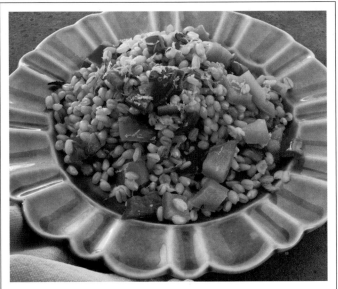

- Place wheat berries and water in a pot or slow cooker. Simmer for two hours.

- When wheat berries are done, heat 2 tablespoons olive oil into a large frying pan over medium heat.

- Add onion, peppers, celery, fennel, and orange zest, and sauté.

- After about 4 minutes, when the vegetables are softened, remove from heat. Mix the cooked wheat berries with vegetables, and serve as a side dish.

Hearty wheat berry salad: If you marinate the cooked wheat berries in a vinaigrette, the acid in the marinade will soften the berries. Combine 1 cup cooked wheat berries in a container with ⅓ cup red wine vinegar and ½ cup olive oil. Add 1 smashed garlic clove and a dash each of oregano, salt, and pepper. Cover and refrigerate overnight. Place over crispy greens for a hearty salad the next day.

Wheat berry veggie soup: Add 1 cup cooked wheat berries to 1 quart leftover turkey soup. Add 1 cup cut-up tomatoes, 1 cup sliced carrots, a sliced parsnip, and a few small blue nose turnips cut into small a dice. Soup's on! Serve some crusty slices of toasted multigrain bread and a green salad, and dinner's ready.

Rinse Wheat Berries

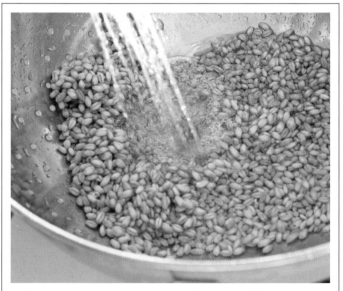

Wheat Berries Instead of Chips

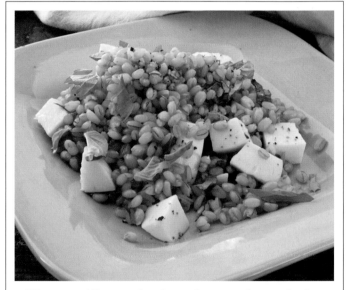

- It's important to rinse wheat berries because they have been harvested in a dirty field and may have a dirt crust on the outside.

- If you don't rinse the berries, the dirt will totally destroy the flavor of your meal.

- Or, you may find a nugget of dirt, which will dissolve under running water.

- What a treat! Set out a bowl of wheat berries drenched in vinaigrette with fresh basil and small chunks of low-fat mozzarella.

- For color, add 1 cup quartered cherry tomatoes and cubed green bell peppers.

- Scoop up the goodies by the spoonful on some thin slices of multigrain bread.

HIGH-FIBER FOODS

CHICKEN CURRY WITH RICE

You can make this curry in a hurry and please everyone's taste, from hot to mild

When you start to understand Indian cooking, you'll find that there is not just one spice blend that is the "curry." An experienced chef will mix his or her spices to suit the dish, the occasion, and the personal tastes of family and guests.

For the purposes of this recipe, get a premium blend of Madras curry powder from your supermarket. You can always add hot chilies or cayenne pepper to increase the heat.

There are probably a thousand recipes for chicken curry. This one is quite easy and delicious. It's a wonderful party dish, as you can make a big batch in advance and keep it warm on a hot tray. Serve with rice and lots of garnishes on the side. *Yield: 8 servings*

Ingredients

1 tablespoon cooking oil, such as canola or peanut

2 pounds chicken tenders (defrosted if frozen), cut into 1-inch pieces

1 cup chopped onion

2 green chilies, cored and finely minced (optional)

2 cloves garlic, peeled and chopped

1 tablespoon curry powder, or to taste

1 tablespoon fresh gingerroot, peeled and minced

$1/2$ cup canned low-fat condensed cream-of-chicken soup

$1/2$ cup unsweetened coconut milk

$1/4$ cup chicken broth

2 tablespoons ground cashews

4 cups cooked brown rice

Calories 454, **Fat** (g) 17, **Carbohydrates** (g) 41, **Protein** (g) 34, **Fiber** (g) 4, **Saturated Fat** (g) 7, **Cholesterol** (mg) 76, **Sodium** (mg) 403, **Carb Choices** 3, **ADA Exchange** 3 starch, 3 medium-fat meat

Chicken Curry with Rice

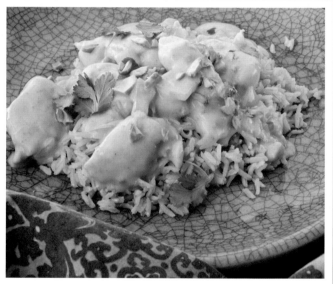

- Heat oil in a large pan. Sauté chicken pieces; when golden brown on both sides, remove from pan and set aside.

- Add onion, optional chilies, and garlic; cook 5 to 7 minutes to soften. Stir in curry powder and blend well. Blend in gingerroot.

- Add remaining ingredients and stir, cooking over very low heat.

- Return chicken to pan; simmer another 10 minutes. Serve with rice.

Garnishes for curry: Curry is enhanced by a number of garnishes. Bowls of cashews and peanuts are excellent. Cucumbers, chopped and marinated in lemony yogurt, make a refreshing side. A bowl of fresh pineapple chunks is cooling, as are orange slices.

• • • • RECIPE VARIATION • • • •

Fresh apple chutney: Use 1 cup cored, chopped apples (leave the skin on for color), ¼ cup chopped onion, 1 teaspoon fresh ginger, 2 tablespoons apple cider vinegar, 1 teaspoon Splenda, ⅛ teaspoon ground cloves, and ⅛ teaspoon chili powder, more or less to taste. Make it a day in advance; marinate the chicken, covered, in the refrigerator. Substitute peaches or mangos for apples.

Working with Chicken Tenders

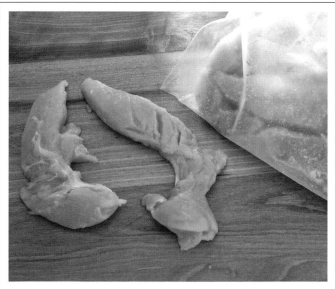

- Chicken tenders are a gift to any busy cook. They can go from freezer to pot with no fuss and in little time.

- They are excellent for people with diabetes and dieters, as they are skinless and lower in fat and calories.

- Cut them into strips for stir-fry, or into chunks for a quick addition to pasta sauce.

- Or, make a chicken potpie with loads of vegetables and chicken tenders.

Adjusting Heat in Curry

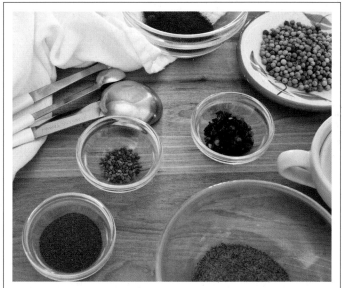

- Adjust the heat of a curry dish by adding or removing pepper.

- Lightly colored curries often use white pepper.

- The heat in curry can come from a number of sources, including cayenne (ground red pepper), red pepper flakes, chili powder, black pepper, fresh chilies, and hot paprika.

- Therefore, you can make your curry as hot or as mild as you wish. Remember, fresh chilies should be handled with care, as they can burn your skin.

SZECHWAN BEEF WITH VEGETABLES

Stir-fried beef with vegetables is a staple in many Chinese restaurants

This recipe features strips of filet mignon marinated briefly to add flavor. The fillet needs very little cooking.

Once you get into stir-frying and using a wok, you will absolutely depend on it for quick and diverse meals.

A good, stainless-steel wok is an excellent addition to any kitchen. If the bottom is copper clad, that's even better, and it should come with a collar to hold it in place on your stove.

You can use sugar snap or snow peas, bamboo shoots, and/or any variety of bean sprouts. Frozen baby peas are also very good, and scallions are an essential part of any stir-fry.

Making a delicious marinade that's also used in cooking saves time, something we all appreciate. *Yield: 6 servings*

Ingredients

For the marinade/sauce:

¹/₄ cup light soy sauce

2 teaspoons garlic powder

¹/₂ teaspoon Chinese five-spice powder

¹/₂ teaspoon ground coriander seeds

1 teaspoon ground black pepper

2 tablespoons Asian sesame seed oil

1 pound filet mignon, fat removed and cut into strips, 1 inch long and ¹/₂ inch wide

For the vegetables:

1 tablespoon canola oil

¹/₂ pound sugar snap peas, ends trimmed

1 6-ounce can water chestnuts, drained, rinsed, and cut into halves

1 bunch scallions, cut into 1-inch pieces

¹/₂ cup beef broth

Calories 358, **Fat** (g) 19, **Carbohydrates** (g) 18, **Protein** (g) 29, **Fiber** (g) 3, **Saturated Fat** (g) 4, **Cholesterol** (mg) 82, **Sodium** (mg) 744, **Carb Choice** 1, **ADA Exchange** 1 starch, 3½ medium-fat meat

Szechwan Beef with Vegetables

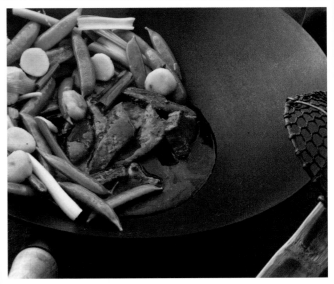

- Whisk sauce ingredients in a large bowl. Add beef; marinate 20 to 30 minutes.

- Pour oil into wok over medium-high heat. Add veggies; cook 2 minutes, stirring often. Push veggies up onto the sides of the wok to slow cooking process.

- Using a slotted spoon to drain marinade, add beef to the wok. Stir-fry beef in wok 2 minutes.

- Stir in beef broth, remaining marinade. Reduce heat; cook, stirring (1 more minute for rare, 1½ minutes for medium, or 3 minutes for well-done).

• • • • RECIPE VARIATION • • • •

Try this Asian-inspired variation: Start with the basic recipe, and just before serving add the following: ½ cup chopped pineapple and ¼ cup sweet red pepper, roasted, peeled, and chopped (from a jar is fine). Roasted unsalted peanuts (¼ cup) add crunch and flavor.

A second variation is to add 1 tablespoon tangerine or clementine zest to the basic recipe, and sprinkle the chopped fruit of 2 tangerines or clementines on the dish just before serving. You can use coriander leaf (cilantro), which is an herb that adds a strong flavor spike. Try adding 2 tablespoons fresh, chopped coriander leaves. But remember, some people are allergic to cilantro, while some just hate it.

Seasoning a Wok

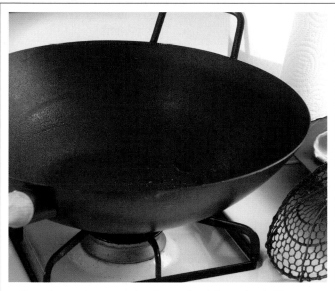

- Now that woks are made of stainless steel, seasoning them is not necessary. However, if your wok isn't stainless, here's how to do it:

- Place cooking oil, preferably one with a high flash point, such as grapeseed oil, in the wok and turn heat on low.

- Let it heat slowly. Then turn off heat, and let the wok sit 30 to 60 minutes.

- Wipe out the wok with a paper towel, and use the wok as often as possible. Cooking in it renews the seasoning.

Cutting Scallions

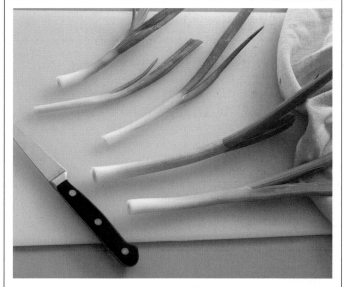

- When chopping a bunch of scallions, first cut off the roots.

- Then, using a sharp paring knife, slit the papery skin remaining at the root end. Peel off the skin and discard.

- The white part of the scallion is full of flavor and can be minced.

- Use a pair of scissors to cut the green parts of the scallion to desired lengths.

PORK SOUVLAKI

Marinated pork is grilled on skewers with onions and bell peppers

Souvlaki is the Greek word for "skewer." It consists of meats and vegetables threaded onto a skewer and grilled until brown and juicy.

Kalamaki (or little reed) is made up of meat cut into small cubes and skewered on wooden skewers. Either way, the meat is marinated in a mixture of lemon, garlic, olive oil, wine, and lots of herbs.

Lamb is traditionally used for this recipe, but you can use pork, chicken breasts, or chicken thighs. The meat is always boneless and is marinated before grilling.

Serve souvlaki with tzatziki sauce, made from sour cream or yogurt and cucumber, a rice pilaf flavored with oregano and mint, a cucumber and tomato salad, and lemon meringue pie. *Yield: 8 servings*

KNACK DIABETES COOKBOOK

Ingredients

1 lemon

3 tablespoons olive oil

2 tablespoons balsamic vinegar

2 tablespoons red wine

1 teaspoon dill weed

1/4 teaspoon dried mint leaves

1/4 teaspoon pepper

1 tablespoon fresh oregano

2 pounds pork tenderloin

2 red onions

3 green bell peppers

Calories 190, **Fat** (g) 10, **Carbohydrates** (g) 4, **Protein** (g) 20, **Fiber** (g) 1, **Saturated Fat** (g) 3, **Cholesterol** (mg) 62, **Sodium** (mg) 20, **ADA Exchange** 3 lean meat

Pork Souvlaki

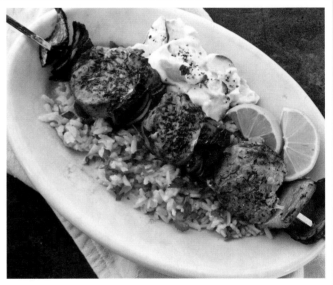

- Prepare grill. Juice lemon; remove zest. Combine juice, zest, olive oil, vinegar, wine, dill, mint, pepper, and oregano in a bowl.

- Cut pork into 1½-inch cubes and add to marinade. Cover and chill 8 to 24 hours.

- Remove pork from marinade; reserve marinade. Cut each onion into eight wedges; cut bell peppers into strips. Thread food onto skewers.

- Grill 6 inches from medium coals 12 to15 minutes. Brush with marinade until pork registers 155°F. Discard remaining marinade. Serve with tzatziki sauce.

• • • • RECIPE VARIATION • • • •

Tzatziki sauce: Peel a cucumber and cut in half; remove seeds. Shred half of the cucumber; drain on paper towels. Mix with 1 cup low-fat sour cream, 2 tablespoons lemon juice, 2 minced cloves of garlic, 1 tablespoon fresh dill weed, and ¼ teaspoon pepper. Serve with souvlaki.

Lamb souvlaki: Make recipe as directed, except use 2 pounds of lean lamb shoulder instead of pork tenderloin. Omit dried mint; add 1 tablespoon minced fresh mint leaves. Omit balsamic vinegar; add 2 tablespoons orange juice. Marinate as directed and grill as directed.

Prepare Marinade

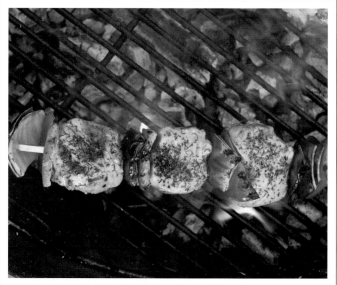

- This marinade recipe is quite variable and forgiving. You can use lime juice instead, add garlic, or omit the mint.

- Use other fresh herbs, omit the balsamic vinegar, and add hot minced chili peppers.

- You can make the marinade ahead of time. Store it in the refrigerator for up to 2 days.

- If you change the marinade and love the results, be sure to write down your formula. Soon, you'll have a notebook full of tried-and-true recipes.

Thread on Skewers

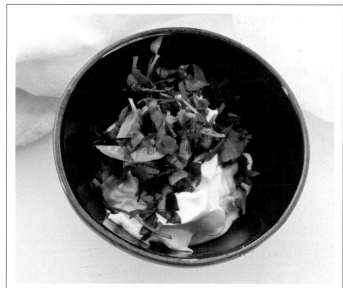

- Metal skewers are the best choice for this type of recipe because the food grills longer than 7 to 8 minutes.

- The onions may be a bit difficult to skewer. If so, use a sharp knife to start a hole.

- You can assemble the skewers ahead of time; cover and refrigerate up to 8 hours.

- It's okay to marinate the pork longer than 24 hours; the meat will be very flavorful and tender.

VEAL STEW WITH CAPERS

Veal makes a most amiable stew, as it gets along happily with almost anything you add

Chunks of veal from the shoulder or flank are considered stew meat. Veal cut from the leg, or chops from the loin or rib, are a lot less expensive than veal cutlets. You can serve veal stew over brown rice or mashed potatoes, with multigrain noodles, or with some crusty French bread for dipping.

Veal is the meat of the calf; its dam is a cow, and its sire is a bull. When you buy veal, look for meat with a pale pink color. If it's red, it's beef.

Traditionally, veal and peppers in tomato sauce are the basic ingredients of an Italian stew. This recipe is a combination of French and Italian influences. Capers are popular in all of the Mediterranean countries. *Yield: 6 servings*

KNACK DIABETES COOKBOOK

Ingredients

¹/₄ cup whole-wheat flour

¹/₄ teaspoon salt

Freshly ground black pepper to taste

1 teaspoon dried oregano

1 teaspoon dried basil

1 teaspoon dried rosemary

1¹/₄ pounds veal stew meat

1 tablespoon olive or canola oil

1 onion, peeled and chopped

1 carrot, peeled and chopped

2 cloves garlic, peeled and chopped

¹/₂ teaspoon Worcestershire sauce

¹/₂ cup dry white wine

¹/₂ cup chicken broth

2 tablespoons capers

¹/₂ bunch fresh parsley, rinsed and coarsely chopped

Calories 160, **Fat** (g) 5, **Carbohydrates** (g) 7, **Protein** (g) 21, **Fiber** (g) 1, **Saturated Fat** (g) 1, **Cholesterol** (mg) 79, **Sodium** (mg) 414, **ADA Exchange** 3 very lean meat, 1 vegetable

Veal Stew with Capers

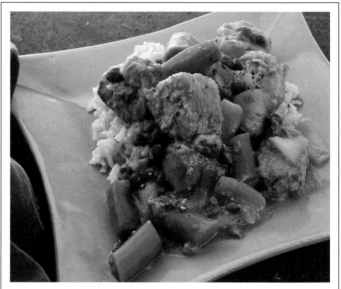

- On a piece of waxed paper, mix flour, salt, pepper, and herbs. Roll stew meat in the flour mixture.

- Heat oil in a large pan over medium heat. Add veal, and brown on all sides. Push to one side of the pan, and add onion, carrot, and garlic.

- Sauté 4 minutes, stirring occasionally. Slowly blend in Worcestershire sauce, wine, broth, and capers. Reduce heat and cover.

- Simmer 1 hour or until very tender. Sprinkle with parsley. Serve with brown rice or whole-grain noodles (optional).

• • • • RECIPE VARIATION • • • •

French veal stew: Veal stew cooks more quickly than beef or lamb stew. White wine will tenderize the stew meat, especially if you marinate it for a couple of hours. You can serve this as a provincial French stew with 2 cans drained and rinsed white beans and lots of herbes de Provence. Simply sauté 2 cleaned and chopped red peppers with 1 whole peeled and chopped onion along with the veal, then add 2 cups of a garlicky tomato sauce to the pan; cover and simmer for 1 to 2 hours. Since the stew cooks for at least an hour, it's smart to make a double recipe and freeze half. When you defrost it, you can add 1 cup of sliced, sautéed mushrooms. Brown mushrooms have more flavor than white ones.

Thickening Your Stew or Soup

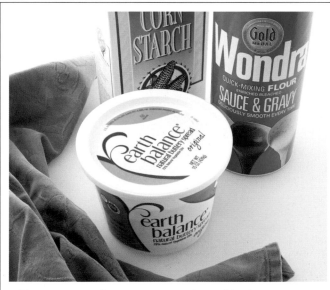

- There are several ways to thicken a stew or soup. The easiest is to sprinkle fast-blending flour into the hot liquid, stirring constantly.

- Or, make a paste with equal amounts soft butter or low-fat margarine and flour. Mix; drop in a dot at a time, stirring constantly.

- Or combine ⅓ cup cornstarch with ½ cup cold water. Whisk with a fork until there are no lumps. Slowly add hot liquid, stirring, then add to pot.

- Don't add regular raw flour to hot liquid, or you will end up with an unpleasantly lumpy stew or soup.

Turning Your Stew into Soup

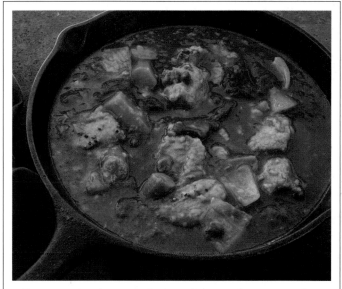

- Turn your stew into soup by adding liquids.

- Two cups of crushed tomatoes, with their juice, will transform your veal stew into soup.

- Chicken broth, wine, or water will also thin your stew and stretch it.

- Stews and soups can also be stretched by the addition of broth, fresh or frozen vegetables such as pearl onions, baby carrots, or zucchini, or a can of red or white beans.

NONA'S MEATBALLS WITH RICOTTA

Adding ricotta cheese to meatballs improves the flavor and texture

This recipe came from Chef Nick Martshenko's grandmother. His *nona* ("grandmother" in Italian) started him on a career that went from the Culinary Institute of America to executive chef at an upscale restaurant.

Martshenko delights customers at Match Restaurant, in Stamford, Connecticut, serving Nona's recipe as an appetizer with tomato sauce and crusty bread. With spaghetti,

it's a great meal. Adding ricotta gives meatballs a rich flavor and nice consistency. Nick's nona used lean ground sirloin, which made the meatballs top-of-the-line. Either round or chuck would also be fine, though chuck is typically a little more fatty. Old-fashioned cooks fry their meatballs, adding a lot of calories from oil. Health-conscious cooks prefer to bake them. *Yield: 8 servings (2 large meatballs per serving)*

Ingredients

1 pound lean ground beef (sirloin, round, or chuck)

1 cup skim-milk ricotta

1 egg

$1/4$ cup grated Parmesan cheese

1 cup fresh soft bread crumbs

$1/4$ teaspoon cinnamon

2 teaspoons dried basil

2 teaspoons dried oregano

Salt and freshly ground black pepper to taste

$1/2$ teaspoon flaxseed or $1/4$ teaspoon aniseed (optional)

1 cup fine bread crumbs

Calories 247, **Fat** (g) 12, **Carbohydrates** (g) 12, **Protein** (g) 21, **Fiber** (g) 1, **Saturated Fat** (g) 5, **Cholesterol** (mg) 62, **Sodium** (mg) 266, **Carb Choice** 1, **ADA Exchange** 1 starch, 2½ medium-fat meat

Nona's Meatballs with Ricotta

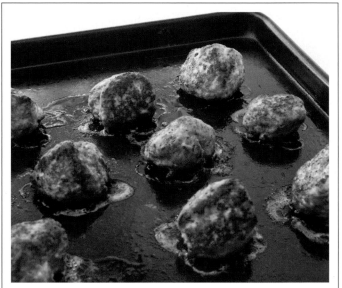

- Preheat oven to 350°F. Combine beef, ricotta, egg, Parmesan, and soft bread crumbs in a large bowl.

- Sprinkle cinnamon, basil, oregano, salt, pepper, and flax- or aniseed over meat mixture. Work mixture until well blended.

- Prepare a baking sheet with nonstick spray, or line it with parchment paper. Make meatballs, rolling them between your palms. Roll them in dry bread crumbs; place on sheet.

- Bake 35 to 40 minutes or until well done and nicely browned.

188

• • • • RECIPE VARIATION • • • •

Spicy and sweet suggestions: Combining beef, pork, and veal is one way to vary this recipe. Substitute ground turkey to reduce calories. With turkey, add ½ cup dried cranberries or raisins. A ½ cup of chopped dried apricots, soaked 30 minutes until plump, give your meatballs a Moroccan touch, along with ½ teaspoon cinnamon added to the mixture. Adding ½ pound fresh sweet or hot Italian sausage gives meatballs a rich, spicy flavor.

Fun variations: The addition of ½ cup pine nuts changes texture considerably. A ½ cup minced fennel bulb gives meatballs a bit of crunch. Use fine crumbs from a multigrain French-style baguette. Serve meatballs over raw or lightly sautéed baby spinach to enhance the nutritional value.

Frying Meatballs

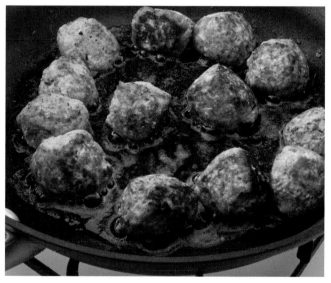

- To fry meatballs, pour 1 inch of oil, such as canola, grapeseed, or peanut, into a frying pan.

- If you use a deep-fat fryer with a basket, you will need more oil. But don't fill it too full; the oil bubbles up and expands when hot.

- Bring oil temperature to 350°F. Don't add meatballs all at once; start with two, bring oil back to temperature, turn meatballs over, and add two more.

- When completely browned, drain meatballs on paper towels, turning so that oil drains off.

Storing Meatballs

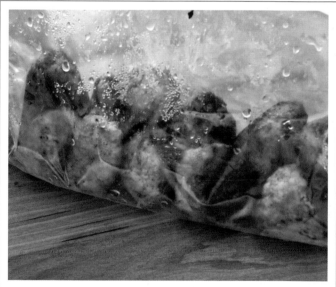

- If you are going to store unsauced meatballs, whether baked or fried, first let them cool.

- Place them on an aluminum foil–covered cookie sheet, making sure they are not touching.

- Freeze meatballs solid.

- Put them in a resealable plastic bag and store in the freezer, using them as needed.

MEDITERRANEAN CASSEROLE

This is a healthy take on paella, the famous Spanish dish made with rice and seafood

For this recipe, you certainly can use frozen shrimp as opposed to fresh. A few pieces of chicken are also a very good addition, and you can substitute fresh or frozen scallops for the shrimp. All of the seafood, chicken, and sausage add flavor to the rice as it absorbs the cooking juices. Herbs and saffron will make your baked rice dish very special. Although saffron is the most expensive spice in the world, it's worth it for a special-occasion dinner.

A garniture of chopped green olives, capers, or green peppercorns will enhance the dish. *Yield: 8 servings*

KNACK DIABETES COOKBOOK

Ingredients

¹/₄ cup olive oil

1 small chicken, cut into **8** pieces

Freshly ground black pepper

Sprinkle of fast-blending flour

1 medium-size onion, peeled and chopped

2 cloves garlic, peeled and chopped

1 sweet green or red pepper, cored, seeded and diced

¹/₄ pound chorizo sausage, cut into ¹/₄-inch coins

2 cups short-grain rice

2 cups chicken broth

1 cup dry white wine

2 cups clam broth or water

¹/₂ teaspoon turmeric

¹/₂ teaspoon cumin

1 tablespoon oregano

¹/₂ teaspoon saffron

32 littleneck clams

32 cleaned mussels

32 jumbo shrimp, raw, peeled, and deveined

Calories 442, **Fat** (g) 14, **Carbohydrates** (g) 46, **Protein** (g) 30, **Fiber** (g) 0, **Saturated Fat** (g) 3, **Cholesterol** (mg) 97, **Sodium** (mg) 366, **Carb Choices** 3, **ADA Exchange** 3 starch, 4 lean meat

Mediterranean Casserole

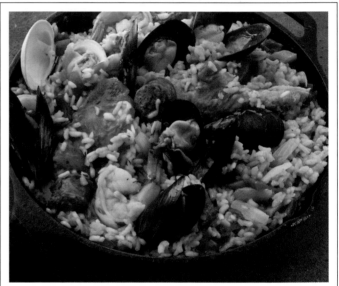

- Preheat oven to 350°F. Heat oil over medium-high heat on stovetop in a large pot.

- Sprinkle chicken with pepper and flour. Sauté 5 minutes, turning to brown both sides. Add onion, garlic, and peppers. Sauté, stirring occasionally, for 8 minutes. Mix in sausage.

- Blend in rice and cook, stirring, 5 to 6 minutes. Pour in liquids, ½ cup at a time, stirring. Blend seasonings. Bake 15 minutes. Press clams and mussels into rice. Return pot to oven. When rice blooms, add shrimp, pressing into rice mixture. Cook until all shellfish are open and shrimp is pink.

ZOOM

About rice: Rice has been cultivated in Asia for 5,000 years. A staple of Chinese, Indian, Japanese, and Southeast Asian cooking, it sustains huge populations. Rice migrated to Japan, India, and the Middle East from China. Then, it made a short trip across the Mediterranean to Europe. In the 1800s, slave owners brought skilled Africans from Angola and settled them on islands off the coast of the Carolinas to grow rice. Brown rice is unpolished and less processed than white rice. It has more fiber, texture, vitamins, and minerals as well. Quick-cooking rice is highly processed. Although it takes only a minute to make, you lose some flavor, nutrition, and texture.

Know When the Rice Is Done

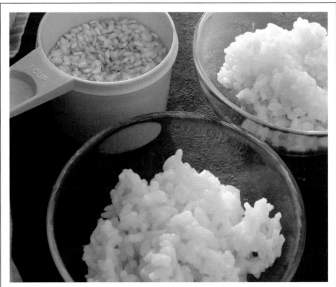

- Rice should not be al dente; you don't want anyone to crack a tooth. You don't want mushy or burned rice, either.

- The easiest way to check the doneness of rice is to take a teaspoonful and taste it.

- Rice actually "blooms," which means that it expands, absorbing the flavors in the broth and seasonings.

- If the rice is not done but is drying out, pour in a bit more liquid and continue cooking.

The Order of Addition

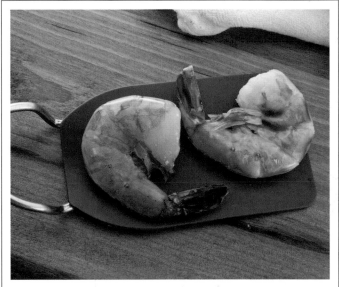

- When adding seafood to a dish, you don't want to overcook or undercook it.

- Overcooked shrimp has the texture of rubber. The same goes for scallops, which need very little cooking.

- An underdone clam or mussel is not opened. Give it more heat; discard any shellfish that does not open. If a shrimp is pink on one side and gray on the other, turn it over.

- Seafood must always be carefully watched. It's too easy to ruin and too expensive to waste.

TINY TURKEY MEATBALLS

These are excellent for an afterschool snack or for adults in a hurry

There is so much more to turkey than Thanksgiving dinner. It's low in fat, high in protein, and can be the base for everything from meatballs to chili.

This is a simple recipe. It is easy to make, baked, and very nutritious. People should eat a small amount of food frequently; eating a little bit helps to keep blood sugar steady, avoiding metabolic highs and lows. For dieters, snacks keep energy levels high and prevent the body from going into "starvation mode." Neither situation is good for any human being.

Don't skip a meal; eat a little, eat often, and eat healthy.

Yield: 32 small meatballs; serving size, 3 meatballs

Ingredients

For the meatballs:

1 egg

1/2 teaspoon ground black pepper, or to taste

1/2 teaspoon hot pepper sauce, or to taste

1 teaspoon salt

1 teaspoon cumin

1 teaspoon garlic powder, or to taste

1/4 teaspoon cinnamon

1 tablespoon tomato paste

1 pound ground turkey

1/2 cup seasoned bread crumbs

1/4 cup raisins

1 tablespoon ground walnuts

For the coating:

1 egg

1/2 teaspoon Tabasco sauce

1 teaspoon chili sauce

1 1/2 cups multigrain cereal, ground in food processor

Calories 127, **Fat** (g) 5, **Carbohydrates** (g) 12, **Protein** (g) 9, **Fiber** (g) 1, **Saturated Fat** (g) 2, **Cholesterol** (mg) 54, **Sodium** (mg) 414, **ADA Exchange** 1 starch, 1 medium-fat meat

Tiny Turkey Meatballs

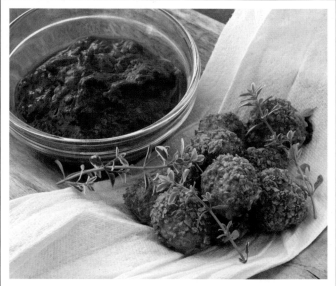

- Preheat oven to 350°F. Prepare a large baking pan with nonstick spray.

- Whisk together the first eight ingredients. Work in the ground turkey and bread crumbs. Mix in raisins and nuts. Form 32 small meatballs, about 1 inch in diameter.

- Whisk egg, Tabasco, and chili sauce together. Roll meatballs in egg mixture, then in crushed cereal.

- Place meatballs in prepared baking pan. Bake 35 minutes, or until well browned. Cool.

• • • • RECIPE VARIATION • • • •

Enriching the meatballs: Meat from the drumstick and thigh of turkey is richer, moister, and somewhat more caloric than white breast meat. Supermarkets sell both dark- and white-meat ground turkey. Enrich basic turkey meatballs with ¼ cup finely chopped toasted walnuts, raisins, currants, or pine nuts. Throw in an extra egg white, ¼ cup milk, and 1 ounce Parmesan cheese.

Coating Your Meatballs

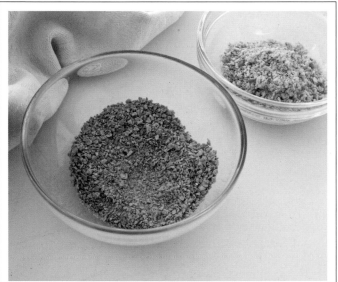

- There are many good coatings for meatballs, which should have a nice, crisp crust. Making your own crumbs from multigrain bread is ideal.

- Commercial crumbs are fine, but read labels for seasonings and salt.

- Ground crackers are usually too salty to be good for people with diabetes. Most cereals are too sweet.

- Crumbled homemade corn bread produces an excellent coating, but you have to retoast the bread after you've made crumbs.

Shaping Meatballs

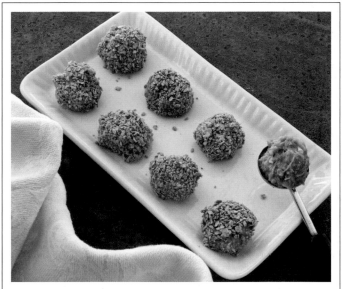

- Toss the meat, crumbs, and other ingredients with two forks.

- If you pat the meat and roll it too tightly, it will be denser than desired.

- Try using a melon ball scoop to make meatballs of equal size, which is important for uniform baking.

193

MINI-WAFFLE SPREAD

This low-fat treat is perfect for kids as well as adults with a sweet tooth

It's important for kids and adults alike to snack on foods that will nourish and provide energy without adding sugar or fat to their diets. Obesity in children is linked to early-onset type 2 diabetes. Adults can provide great workplace snacks for the family with little effort.

Low-fat cottage cheese is an excellent base for many flavorful spreads. The spark of a tart apple, the crunch of nuts, and a touch of Splenda, cinnamon, or nutmeg will give you a spread that goes on mini waffles or crackers. Cheese adds calcium, and fruit and nuts add fiber and other nutrients. Keep a half pint of the spread at work and another half pint at home for snacking. *Yield: 12 ounces, (1 ounce per serving)*

Ingredients

¹/₂ pint (8 ounces) low-fat, small-curd cottage cheese

3 tablespoons chopped, toasted walnuts

1 small tart apple, cored and chopped, skin on

Juice of ¹/₂ lemon

1 teaspoon Splenda

¹/₂ teaspoon cinnamon

Pinch of nutmeg

Toasted mini waffles from the freezer as needed (multigrain waffles recommended)

Calories 20, **Fat** (g) 0, **Carbohydrates** (g) 2, **Protein** (g) 2, **Fiber** (g) 0, **Saturated Fat** (g) 0, **Cholesterol** (mg) 1, **Sodium** (mg) 111, **ADA Exchange** free food

Mini-Waffle Spread

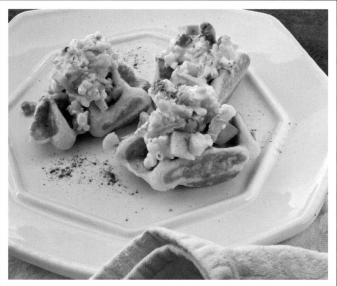

- Mix cottage cheese and nuts in a bowl.

- In a separate bowl, sprinkle chopped apple with lemon juice to prevent the apple from browning.

- Work Splenda and spices into the cheese; mix in apple pieces. Store in an airtight container, and refrigerate leftover spread.

- Prepare mini waffles according to package directions. Top each waffle with 1 teaspoon of spread.

Fruits and nuts: Vary the types of fruits and nuts you add to the low-fat cottage cheese. A half cup chopped toasted almonds, pecans, or peanuts are fine. Just make sure that they are not salted. Any fruit you like can be substituted for apples. Try it with chopped fresh figs for a terrific treat. From sweet to savory: Transform this sweet treat into a savory one by omitting the sugar and adding 1 tablespoon Parmesan or Gorgonzola cheese. A half cup finely chopped radishes, carrots, celeriac, fennel, or celery is also a wonderful addition, with negligible calories. Dried or fresh herbs to add for a savory combination include 1 tablespoon either basil, oregano, rosemary, or thyme. Lots of black pepper is another good addition.

How to Mix Successfully

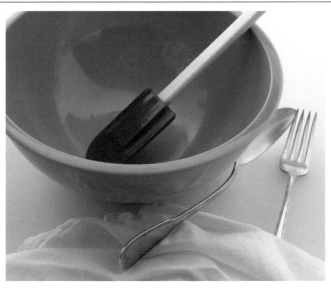

- The last thing you want is to bite into a concentrated lump of Splenda or find that all of the cinnamon has landed in one place.

- The best way to blend the cheese with the sugar and spice is to premix them in a bowl with a fork.

- Using a rubber scraper, mix from the outside in.

- Repeat the process until well blended, then add the apple.

Roasting and Toasting Nuts

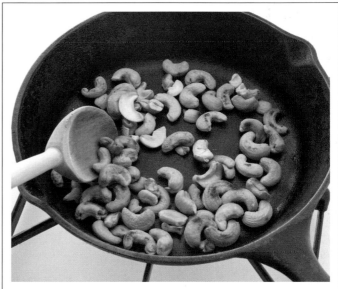

- There are basically two ways to roast and toast nuts.

- One is to do it in a hot skillet, preferably a heavy-bottomed, cast-iron frying pan. As soon as the pan is hot, add the nuts; keep them moving and turn often.

- Another method is to bake them in a 325°F oven for 10 to 15 minutes.

- Running them under the broiler is dangerous—it's all too easy to burn the nuts, even if you only look away for a second.

PIZZA WITH ZUCCHINI & CHEESE

You can't go wrong with a healthful, delicious pizza, topped with zucchini and low-fat cheese

Making a truly healthful, low-fat pizza is not all that hard. For this recipe, use low-fat whipped cream cheese in place of mozzarella or mascarpone, a rich and very creamy cheese that's loaded with calories.

Low-fat cream cheese is fat reduced, and lots of flavor is gained with the addition of a bit of Parmesan. Oregano, red pepper flakes, and a bit of extra-virgin olive oil will give your pizza a lot of zing.

You can put as many different vegetables on a "white" pizza (one without tomato sauce) as you would on a "red" pizza. Specialty stores carry multigrain and whole-wheat pizza dough, freshly made and ready to use. *Yield: 12 small snack-size servings*

Ingredients

16 ounces fresh pizza dough, preferably multigrain or whole wheat

Extra-virgin olive oil, in a spray bottle or mister

4 ounces low-fat whipped cream cheese, at room temperature

1 teaspoon dried oregano

1 teaspoon red pepper flakes, or to taste

1/4 cup finely grated Parmesan cheese

1 large or 2 medium-size zucchini, sliced very thin

Calories 192, **Fat** (g) 10, **Carbohydrates** (g) 20, **Protein** (g) 6, **Fiber** (g) 3, **Saturated Fat** (g) 1, **Cholesterol** (mg) 6, **Sodium** (mg) 293, **Carb Choice** 1, **ADA Exchange** 1 starch, 1 vegetable, 2 fat

Pizza with Zucchini & Cheese

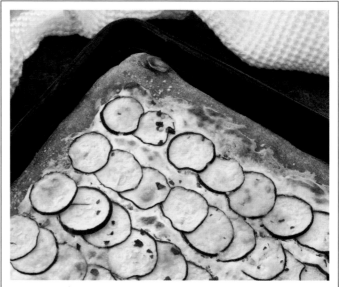

- Preheat oven to 425°F. Prepare a cookie sheet with nonstick spray.

- Roll dough into a 9x12-inch rectangle, and press it down on the cookie sheet. Spray it lightly with olive oil.

- Spread dough with cream cheese; sprinkle with oregano, red pepper flakes, and half the Parmesan.

- Arrange zucchini slices over top. Sprinkle with the remaining cheese, and give it another misting of olive oil. Bake 14 to 16 minutes, or until crust is golden brown.

•••• RECIPE VARIATION ••••

Lots and lots of veggies: Vary this basic pizza with other veggies. Try substituting 1 cup chopped, cooked broccoli rabe for zucchini. A cup of precooked, chopped broccoli also makes a wonderful topping. Or try 1 cup packed fresh baby spinach leaves spread on the pizza, but be sure to give it a good spritz of olive oil.

Cheese variations: There's no reason why you can't make pizzas with different cheeses. No one is "stuck" with whipped cream cheese, mozzarella, and/or Parmesan. Try using 6 ounces grated Manchego cheese from Spain as an alternative. Gorgonzola is wonderful with broccoli or zucchini. Stay away from the heavy, creamy cheeses, such as Brie, Camembert, and Saga blue. They are loaded with fat. And remember, pizza is a treat, not part of your daily diet.

Arranging Pizza Toppings

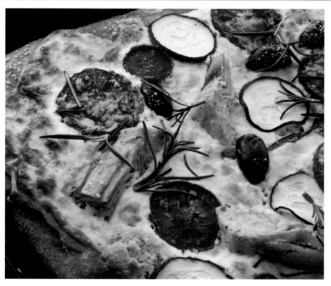

- The top of a pizza can be a work of art or a mess.

- Arranging the toppings artfully takes a bit more time than just throwing stuff on dough. Make a geometric design with zucchini, pepperoni, and/or pepper strips.

- Don't let the cheese clump in one place; sprinkle or spread it evenly.

- If your oven heats unevenly, turn the pizza around when halfway done so that it will brown evenly.

Grinding and/or Grating Cheese

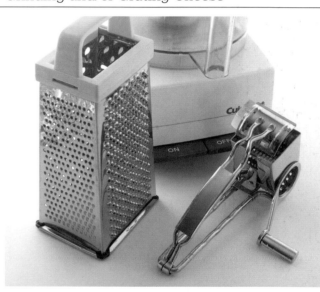

- An old-fashioned box grater does a fine job with semi-soft and even some hard cheeses. You get a coarse grate, which is fine for some dishes.

- For grinding, use either a cheese grinder or the metal blade on your food processor.

- When you attempt to grate or grind soft cheeses, such as mozzarella or Brie, they clump.

- For pizza, a finer grind of Parmesan is better than a coarse one.

CROSTINI WITH MUSHROOMS

Yet another Italian creation, crostini are so much better than ordinary crackers

Crostini can be made large with Italian bread, or small with a baguette. Either way, use multigrain if possible. Freshly baked multigrain breads are available in most supermarkets. The combination of grains results in the crunch and nutty flavor of the bread.

Crostini can be classically topped with garlic, tomato, and basil. Or go wild with toppings. Sautéed mushrooms are lovely when dressed with vinaigrette and spread warm over crostini. Follow your taste preferences. Very low in salt, crostini have almost no sugar, and multigrain varieties have an added value with fiber. Health benefits of crostini far outweigh any commercial cracker. *Yield: 8 servings (4 crostini per serving)*

Ingredients

For the topping:

1 tablespoon olive oil

2 shallots, peeled and minced

1 cup cleaned, chopped mushrooms (shiitake, porcini, or white)

2 tablespoons red wine vinegar

1 teaspoon dried thyme leaves

1 tablespoon low-fat mayonnaise

$1/4$ cup finely grated Parmesan cheese

For the crostini:

1 multigrain baguette, about 8 inches long

Olive oil, in a spray bottle or mister

1 tablespoon garlic powder

1 tablespoon dried oregano

Calories 137, **Fat** (g) 5, **Carbohydrates** (g) 17, **Protein** (g) 6, **Fiber** (g) 1, **Saturated Fat** (g) 2, **Cholesterol** (mg) 6, **Sodium** (mg) 283, **Carb Choice** 1, **ADA Exchange** 1 starch, 1 fat

Crostini with Mushrooms

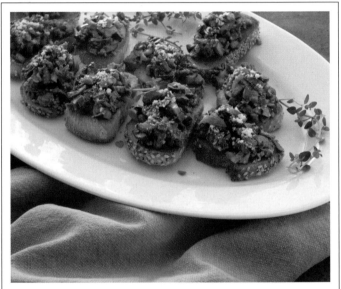

- Heat oil in a frying pan over medium-high heat. Sauté shallots and mushrooms until softened, about 10 minutes. Add vinegar, thyme, and mayonnaise; let cool. Sprinkle with cheese.

- Preheat oven to 400°F. Prepare a cookie sheet with nonstick spray.

- Cut baguette on a diagonal, ¼ inch per slice. Arrange on cookie sheet; bake until lightly brown. Turn over. Spray with oil; sprinkle with garlic powder, oregano. Bake until crisp and brown.

- Spread each crostini with 1 tablespoon of spread. Serve.

• • • • RECIPE VARIATION • • • •

Diversity in toppings: After you've toasted one side of the crostini, you can put a topping on the other side and bake it a bit longer for a melted treat. Various cheeses are excellent; try 8 ounces of crumbled Gorgonzola or low-fat Swiss mixed with 1 cup chopped, low-salt ham; 1 cup chopped fresh figs; or, as in this recipe, 1 cup mushrooms. Or you can simply spray the untoasted side of the crostini with olive oil; sprinkle with 1 tablespoon each of oregano, garlic powder, and pepper; and toast some more. Crostini are fine plain or served with 2 cups of dip on the side. A half pint of fresh tomatoes, chopped and mixed with basil and diced mozzarella, is very good and can be served hot or cold. If you heat this crostini, the cheese melts. Experiment with goat cheese, olives, figs, and apples as toppings.

Mincing and Chopping

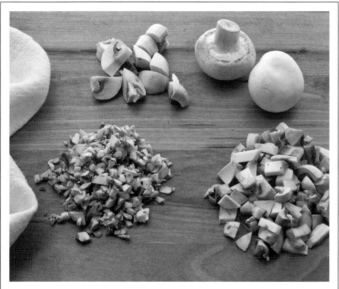

- Mincing is the smallest cut you can make. To mince, you need a chef's knife or a Chinese cleaver.

- The Chinese call this work "march chop" because it makes the sound of a very fast march. When you've chopped all the food in one direction, revolve the chopping board, or move ingredients around and chop them the other way.

- If you use a food processor, keep pulsing it until it reaches the desired size.

- Dicing requires cutting veggies into squares, which range in size.

Bake or Broil?

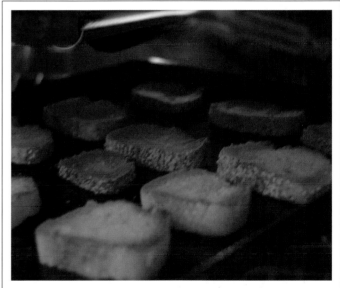

- Under a very hot broiler, one side will be done in about 30 seconds, and the other side in 8 to 10 seconds.

- Baking at 450°F takes slightly less time; the crostini will be a bit crisper if you broil them.

- No matter what you do, watch the crostini—they burn very easily.

- Either way you toast them, don't char the crostini.

199

DEVILED EGGS WITH SHRIMP

A popular snack for decades, here is a healthier version of deviled eggs

Dilled baby shrimp turn deviled eggs into a gourmet treat. Buy the smallest eggs you can find. Medium-size eggs are best for snacking. You may have to settle for large eggs, but do not get extra large or jumbo eggs, or you risk having your snack become a meal.

The "devil" in the eggs can be extremely hot or just a bit spicy.

Mustard is essential, as is mayonnaise, which gives the egg yolks their silky texture. After that, you can mix in all kinds of other ingredients. People love deviled eggs. On most cocktail buffets, deviled eggs are the first items to disappear. Reduce the calories in deviled eggs by using low-fat mayonnaise.

Yield: 6 servings (2 pieces per serving)

KNACK DIABETES COOKBOOK

Ingredients

For the deviled eggs:

6 hard-boiled eggs, cooled and peeled

3 yolks

2 tablespoons low-fat mayonnaise

2 teaspoons prepared yellow mustard or Dijon-style mustard

Salt to taste

Tabasco sauce to taste

For the topping:

1 tablespoon olive oil

Juice of ½ lemon

Salt to taste

Freshly ground black pepper to taste

1 teaspoon dried dill weed

¾ cup baby or salad shrimp, chopped

Calories 136, **Fat** (g) 10, **Carbohydrates** (g) 2, **Protein** (g) 12, **Fiber** (g) 0, **Saturated Fat** (g) 3, **Cholesterol** (mg) 279, **Sodium** (mg) 324, **ADA Exchange** 1½ medium-fat meat, 1 fat

Deviled Eggs with Shrimp

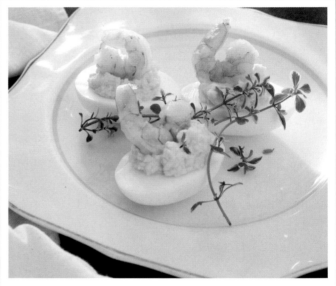

- Cut eggs in half, scoop three yolks into a bowl and arrange whites on a plate.

- Place next four ingredients in food processor and pulse until very smooth. Pause every 10 seconds to scrape sides of bowl.

- Taste for seasoning. You can always make it hotter but not milder.

- Make topping by whisking all but shrimp in bowl. Add shrimp; toss gently to coat.

- Spoon topping over the finished eggs, gently pressing the baby shrimp into the whipped yolks.

•••• RECIPE VARIATION ••••

Endless versatility: When you start with a basic recipe for deviled eggs, there is no limit to what you can add, or the garnishes that transform them every time. By mixing 3 tablespoons minced smoked salmon into the yolks, you will have a whole different egg. Or you can simply place snips of salmon on top. A sprinkling (about ⅛ teaspoon) of red or black caviar is classic and great with champagne for a special party.

Flavoring eggs: Four green peppercorns on top of each egg make them really come alive, as do four capers. A teaspoon of crabmeat salad pressed down into each of the whipped yolks is also very good. Two tablespoons of minced green onions (scallions) added to the yolk mixture are also quite nice, as are snipped fresh chives on top.

How to Hard-Boil Eggs

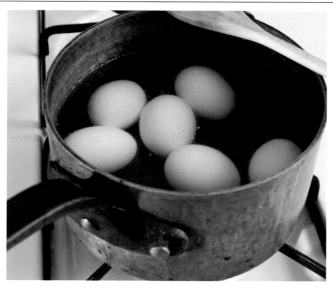

- Place eggs in pot of cold water on stove. Turn the heat on high.

- When the water is scalding hot (small bubbles showing at the edges of the pan), turn the heat to simmer and cover eggs. If you are using a very heavy pot, remove it from the stove.

- Let eggs sit 10 to 12 minutes in hot water.

- Place pot of eggs under cold running water. As soon as you can touch them, crack each egg and return it to the pot of cold water. When all are cracked, peel them.

How to Easily Peel Eggs

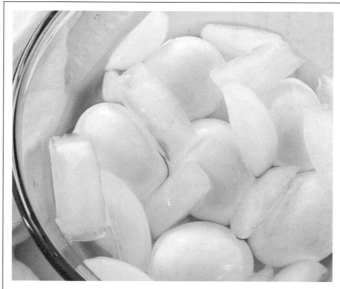

- Sometimes an egg won't peel easily because it's almost too fresh.

- Return it to the boiling water, then plunge it in ice water to shrink the egg.

- If your eggs turn into an irretrievable mess, looking moth-eaten and rough, simply make egg salad, placing the mixture in a bowl, with crackers or crostini on the side. Then add your shrimp garnish for a new "egg-sperience."

CHICKEN WITH PEANUT SAUCE

These chicken tenders can be served hot, cold, or at room temperature

Grilled or broiled, the results are pretty much the same with chicken tenders. When they are marinated and either charcoal-grilled or run under the broiler, they are an excellent and flavorful source of protein.

The tender is the strip across the very top of the chicken breast, and its size reflects the size of the chicken. Tenders are available in bags, fresh or frozen, at your supermarket. A bag of frozen chicken tenders is wonderful to have on hand—it covers you in almost any food emergency. Whether it's the soccer team showing up ravenous after practice, or the bridge club playing at your house, you can make an instant snack that will please everyone. *Yield: 8 servings*

Ingredients

For the chicken:

1/2 cup light soy sauce

1/4 cup fresh or frozen orange juice

1 tablespoon Asian sesame seed oil

1 tablespoon fresh gingerroot, minced

1 1/2 pounds chicken tenders, cut into bite-size pieces

For the sauce:

1/4 cup reduced-fat peanut butter

Juice of 1/2 fresh lime

1 teaspoon fresh gingerroot, minced

3 tablespoons low-sodium soy sauce

Dash of Tabasco or other hot pepper sauce

Calories 155, **Fat** (g) 7, **Carbohydrates** (g) 4, **Protein** (g) 12, **Fiber** (g) 1, **Saturated Fat** (g) 1, **Cholesterol** (mg) 43, **Sodium** (mg) 465, **ADA Exchange** 3 lean meat

Chicken with Peanut Sauce

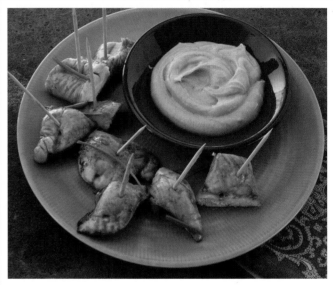

- Whisk the first four ingredients in a bowl; add chicken tenders. Marinate 30 minutes; drain marinade.

- Preheat grill or oven to 400°F. If grilling, thread chicken on eight long skewers. If broiling, place on a pan that you have prepared with nonstick spray.

- Grill or broil tenders until well browned, about 4 minutes per side.

- Whisk sauce ingredients in a bowl. Serve tenders on toothpicks with the sauce handy for dipping.

Chicken tenders can be grilled on skewers over hot coals or run under the broiler. If you are using metal skewers, you don't have to worry about soaking them. If you want to use toothpicks, simply paint the tenders in marinade and broil them. Then, pierce them with toothpicks for easy dipping and eating.

You can add a bit of sugar-free barbecue sauce to the cooked tenders for a snack the kids will love. Or make an easy curry sauce for lunch. Chopped cooked tenders served in wraps are easy to hold and not messy.

Picking Toothpicks and Skewers

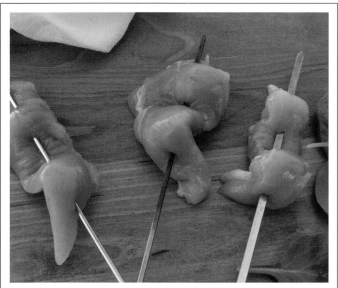

- Never insert plastic toothpicks until after the food has been cooked. Otherwise, the heated plastic will melt into the food.

- If you use wooden toothpicks, soak them prior to cooking, or they will catch fire. It is best, however, to add the toothpicks after tenders are cooked.

- If you are charcoal-grilling tenders, use metal skewers.

- If you are broiling them in the oven, don't bother with skewers; spear them with toothpicks when done.

Switching Up Sizes

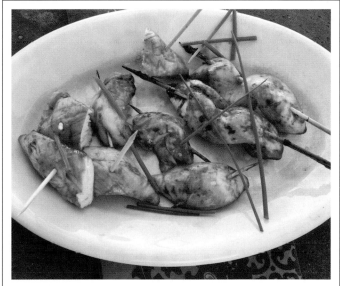

- If you are making the tenders to "grab and go," you probably should make them bite-size.

- When preparing them for a crowd who will be sitting around watching a ball game and eating, make them larger.

- If you are feeding them to little children as a snack, skip the picks and skewers, and serve them as finger food with plenty of paper napkins.

HOMEMADE KETCHUP

Better restaurants make their own ketchup, and now you can, too

Commercial ketchup is usually quite sweet and salty. No one needs all that sugar and sodium. When you make your own, you are in control.

You also will add your own personal touch when you spice up ketchup with sharp vinegar, various types of citrus juice and/or zest, cardamom, and extra cloves, cinnamon, and cumin. Salt and sugar substitutes also work very well.

Make cocktail sauce by adding horseradish and lemon juice to the basic recipe. If you are using the ketchup with burgers, add some beef essence to give it a beefy flavor. Extra Worcestershire sauce is another ingredient that works well when you make your own ketchup. *Yield: 1 quart (32 2-tablespoon servings)*

KNACK DIABETES COOKBOOK

Ingredients

2 28-ounce cans crushed tomatoes or 40 fresh tomatoes, blanched, skinned, and seeded

1/2 cup cider vinegar

1/4 cup Splenda

2 teaspoons cinnamon

6 whole cloves

1 teaspoon garlic powder

1 teaspoon onion powder

1 teaspoon chili powder

1 teaspoon cumin

Salt to taste

1 teaspoon cayenne pepper, or to taste

Homemade Ketchup

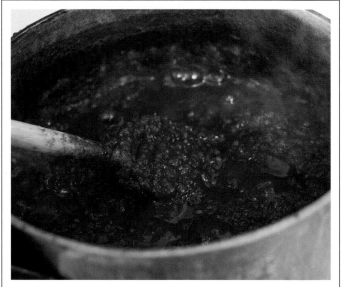

- Mix all the ingredients together in a large saucepan; bring to a boil over medium-high heat.

- Reduce heat to a simmer; cover partially with enough

- venting to let the steam escape, as you want this to cook down.

- Simmer 3 to 4 hours or until your ketchup is thick, rich, and smooth.

Calories 22, **Fat** (g) 0, **Carbohydrates** (g) 5, **Protein** (g) 1, **Fiber** (g) 1, **Saturated Fat** (g) 0, **Cholesterol** (mg) 0, **Sodium** (mg) 21, **ADA Exchange** free exchange

It's easy to transform homemade ketchup into low-salt and low-sugar chili sauce or barbecue sauce. To make chili sauce, start with the basic ketchup recipe. Add 4 ounces tomato paste to the mixture, and cook the mixture down to 3 cups. Add ¼ teaspoon ground cloves and 1 table-spoon Splenda brown sugar.

For barbecue sauce, add 1 tablespoon mustard, extra hot sauce to taste, and a tablespoon molasses. One teaspoon liquid smoke will give your barbecue sauce an outdoor fla-vor even when you are cooking in the oven. If your menu features chicken, try adding 2 ounces raspberry vinegar and 1 ounce orange juice to the sauce.

Blanching Tomatoes

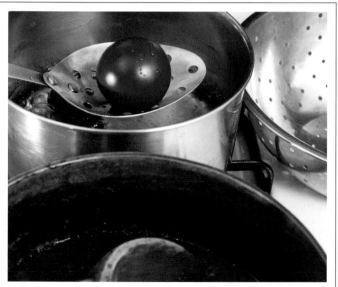

Using Plum Tomatoes

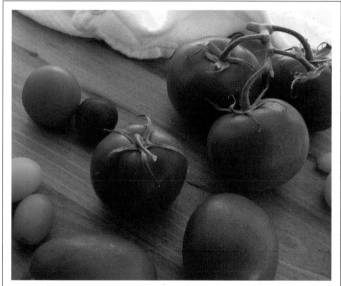

- If you are using fresh toma-toes, you will need to blanch them to remove the skins.

- Prepare a large pot of boiling water, and have a slotted spoon and colander handy.

- Slowly add the tomatoes to the boiling water, keeping track of the order in which you have immersed them. It takes 2 to 3 minutes of cooking to loosen the skins.

- Remove tomatoes to the colander. Allow them to cool, then slip the skins off. Cut out the cores, and chop or grind tomatoes in a food processor.

- Although most tomatoes are available year-round, you will find plum tomatoes in abundance starting in August in most places.

- Plum tomatoes have almost no core, are not very juicy, and have very few seeds. They are dense and meaty.

- They are also called sauce tomatoes or Roma tomatoes.

DRESSINGS, ETC.

HOMEMADE VINAIGRETTE

A basic vinaigrette is always useful and should be on hand at all times

The most basic vinaigrette recipe is elegantly simple: It's a mixture of vinegar and olive oil. The proportion of vinegar to oil varies. It can be ⅓ vinegar to ⅔ oil, or ¼ vinegar to ¾ oil.

The fun part is adding such goodies as minced shallots, basil oil, hot pepper oil, and varying amounts of garlic and herbs. Citrus and fruit vinaigrettes are wonderful with fish and chicken. Fruity ones made with raspberry vinegar are enticing when blended with a fresh peach. Mango and curry vinaigrettes are also excellent options for the creative cook.

Lots of garlic and basil will make a delectable pesto vinaigrette. Add some mint, and use the vinaigrette to dress cold roast lamb for a summer treat. *Yield: 1 cup (8 2-tablespoon servings)*

Ingredients

¹/₄ cup red wine vinegar

2 tablespoons fresh lemon juice

1 teaspoon dry mustard or Dijon-style prepared mustard

¹/₂ teaspoon Worcestershire sauce

1 clove garlic, peeled and mashed

1 shallot, peeled and mashed

1 teaspoon dried oregano, basil, or rosemary (or all three)

Salt and freshly ground black pepper to taste

¹/₂ teaspoon Splenda

¹/₄ cup water

¹/₂ cup extra-virgin olive or canola oil

Calories 83, **Fat** (g) 9, **Carbohydrates** (g) 1, **Protein** (g) 9, **Fiber** (g) 0, **Saturated Fat** (g) 1, **Cholesterol** (mg) 0, **Sodium** (mg) 0, **ADA Exchange** 2 fat

Homemade Vinaigrette

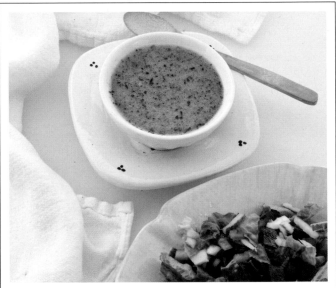

- Place all the ingredients except the water and oil in a food processor.

- Process until well mixed.

- Slowly pour the water and oil into the mixture, pausing to let the oil "digest" the mixture.

- Scrape down the sides of the processor, and give it another whirl. Pour into a glass bottle for serving or short-term storage.

Vinegar variations: Shop specialty aisles and stores, and try to find different vinegars every week. Substitute sherry vinegar from Spain for red wine vinegar. Spanish cuisine is replete with aromatic and delightful sherry vinegar. You can also find pinot grigio and champagne vinegars. Raspberry vinegar is amazing with fruit, as is balsamic vinegar. Simply use as substitutes in the standard recipe.

Oil variations: For Asian flavoring, mix 2 tablespoons sesame seed oil into olive or canola oil. Walnut oil is marvelous as a flavoring added to olive or canola oil. Mix ¼ cup canola oil with ¼ cup olive oil for a light flavor. White truffle oil is delicious. Deduct 1 ounce of canola or olive oil from the basic recipe, and whisk in truffle oil. You can also substitute low-fat mayonnaise for oil to make a creamy dressing.

Whisking vs. Blending

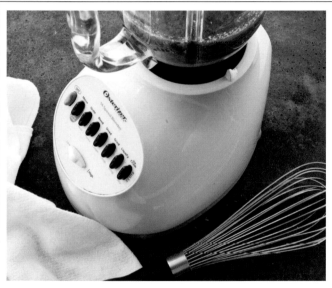

Create Caesar Dressing

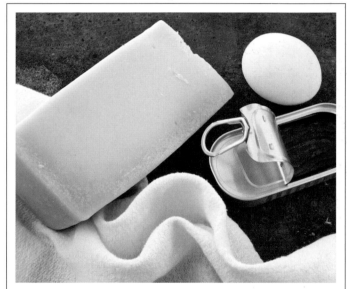

- A wire whisk is the traditional tool for making dressings. Whisking will take longer than using the blender. You will have an entirely unique consistency, as the dressing will separate more easily.

- Blending purees the herbs, fresh or dry, and the aromatic vegetables.

- Use a blender to assure a fully emulsified dressing. And always use a blender for large batches of dressing.

- To create Caesar dressing, add 1 anchovy or ½ inch anchovy paste to the basic vinaigrette recipe and blend well.

- Add 1 raw, pasteurized egg and blend well.

- Pour over 4 servings of prepared romaine lettuce leaves sprinkled with ¼ cup Parmesan cheese.

- Garnish with 2 or 3 low-fat croutons, if desired.

HOMEMADE MUSTARD

This spread can be adjusted to your preference of heat and spice

American mustards are milder than European mustards. In 1814 Jeremiah Colman began processing mustard and was given Queen Victoria's seal of approval. Colman's English Mustard is still around and available in most supermarkets. The powdered mustard is easy to mix into sauces and pastes.

Mustard grows just about everywhere, and the leaves, flowers, and seeds are edible. The three most popular mustard varieties are the black, brown, and white. Yellow food dye is added to the white seeds to color them.

Thousands of years ago, the Greeks and Romans used mustard for medicinal purposes in poultices and dressings. Today, mustard is second only to black pepper in popularity—and now you can make your own. *Yield: ½ cup (24-teaspoon servings)*

Ingredients

¹/₄ cup powdered English mustard

¹/₄ cup cold water

3 tablespoons olive oil

¹/₃ cup white wine or champagne vinegar

¹/₂ teaspoon salt

¹/₂ teaspoon Splenda

¹/₂ teaspoon Tabasco sauce

Optional: ¹/₂ teaspoon celery salt, 1 teaspoon Worcestershire sauce

Calories 49, **Fat** (g) 5, **Carbohydrates** (g) 1, **Protein** (g)1, **Fiber** (g)1, **Saturated Fat** (g) 0, **Cholesterol** (mg) 0, **Sodium** (mg) 99, **ADA Exchange** 1 tablespoon fat

Homemade Mustard

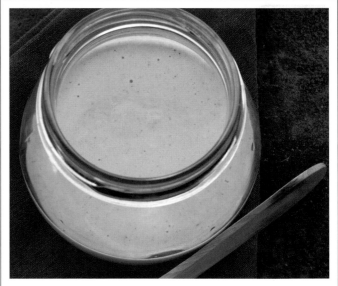

- Using a fork, blend the powdered mustard and cold water until all lumps are gone.

- Pour the mustard and remaining ingredients into a blender, and mix until smooth.

- Taste for seasonings and add more Tabasco, Splenda, salt, vinegar, or optional ingredients as desired.

- Place in a glass jar and store in the refrigerator. It will keep for months.

More on mustard: Most mustard contains honey or sugar. When making mustard at home, sweeten with Splenda. By using a mortar and pestle, it's easy to grind brown, black, or white mustard seeds to as coarse a consistency as you'd like. Mixing mustard powder with various types of vinegar, juice, and wine also creates delightful changes. Mustard is an essential ingredient in many barbecue sauces, pickle relishes, and salad dressings. It is a subtle ingredient in Hollandaise sauce, and essential in mayonnaise and white sauce for fish and chicken. Mustard makes an excellent sauce for beef when mixed with soy sauce, and it's the "devil" in deviled eggs. And what would a hot dog be without mustard?

Grainy Coarse Mustard

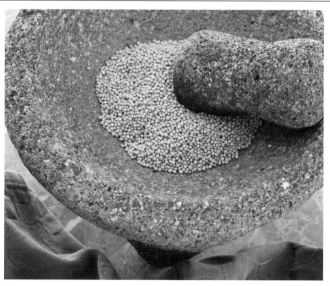

- Mustard seeds are available in many natural food and gourmet shops. Buy 2 ounces at a time.

- Grind the seeds a tablespoon at a time to the desired consistency using a mortar and pestle.

- Follow the above recipe, substituting the freshly ground mustard.

- Store in a jar or crock, and refrigerate.

Changing the Flavor

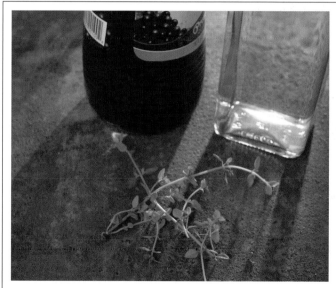

- Vinegar comes in a variety of flavors that you can use to change the flavor of your mustard at will.

- Try substituting ¼ cup sherry or raspberry vinegar for the white. Or, substitute ¼ cup orange juice for the water.

- Another way to change the flavor is to mix lemon zest into your mustard.

- You can add various herbs at will—just keep experimenting with flavors to develop a combination that is very much your own.

FRUIT COULIS
Liven up meat dishes with the addition of a seasonal fruit coulis

Making coulis requires the use of a blender. Historically, chefs put fruit through a fine sieve, and you might have to do that today to remove the seeds of raspberries or blackberries it you use them. Caution: If someone in your circle has digestive issues, he or she may not be able to handle the seeds even after they've been pureed in the blender.

Use any fruit that is in season. Mangos with a bit of lime juice are excellent. Strawberries, blueberries, and blackberries are also possibilities. Peaches are very good and can be used as a sauce on pork or duck.

Fresh fruit is best. Frozen berries are never quite as good as fresh, and canned fruit is too soft for a coulis. *Yield: 1 cup (4 2-ounce servings)*

Ingredients

1 1/2 cups fresh raspberries, rinsed

1 tablespoon Splenda

1/2 teaspoon salt

Optional: 1/2 teaspoon hot pepper sauce, 1 tablespoon fresh rosemary leaves, or 4 fresh mint leaves

Fruit Coulis

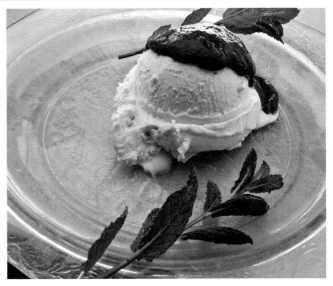

- Pick over the raspberries to make sure there are no stems or bad berries.

- Place all the ingredients in a blender and mix until pureed.

- Add optional ingredients, if desired.

- Store the coulis in a glass jar with a tight-fitting lid in the refrigerator. It will keep for about 1 week.

Calories 24, **Fat** (g) 0, **Carbohydrates** (g) 6, **Protein** (g) 1, **Fiber** (g) 3, **Saturated Fat** (g) 0, **Cholesterol** (mg) 0, **Sodium** (mg) 1, **ADA Exchange** 1 serving equals free food

Savory coulis: By adding spices and/or herbs to the fruit, you will discover a number of creative and wonderful variations. Mixing, as in the recipe below, 1½ cups fresh raspberries with 1 tablespoon fresh rosemary and 1 teaspoon hot sauce or curry powder results in a terrific sauce for duck or chicken. A cup and a half of ripe, cut up pears (skins on) blended with 1 tablespoon lemon juice and 1 cinnamon stick produce a fresh sauce that's delightful on chicken or turkey. Mixing fruit is also an option. Try 3 blanched, peeled, and pitted ripe peaches and ¾ cup raspberries for a melba-type sauce that's as good for dessert as it is with pork or poultry. If you are making a coulis for use with meat or chicken, be sure to use less Splenda; a bit is fine, but you don't want it to be too sweet.

Strain Your Coulis

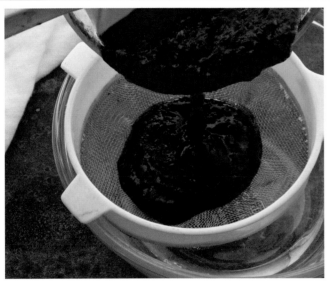

- If you are feeding a person who has denture trouble or certain digestive problems, you may want to strain even the ground-up seeds out of the coulis.

- Simply put the sauce through a fine sieve, stirring with a spoon.

- You may need to add 1 tablespoon hot water to facilitate getting the pulp through the sieve.

- Discard remaining seeds.

Hot Coulis Makes Sauce

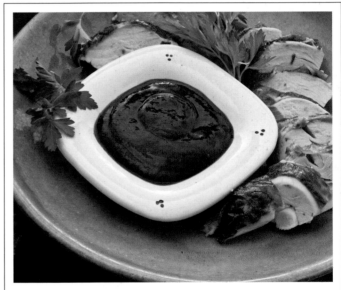

- By heating your coulis, you will transform it from a dessert sauce to one that is very good with meat.

- This technique is adaptable to various flavors of fruit coulis to go with different poultry, meat, or seafood dishes.

- Do not boil it; coulis can burn easily.

- Pour the coulis into the top of a double boiler and heat, keeping the water in the base ½ inch away from the top pot to warm it without burning.

BASIC WHITE SAUCE

There's no limit to what a good cook can do with a basic white sauce

Everyone who cooks needs to know the basics of sauce making. If you can whip up a sauce, you can turn everyday dishes into amazing creations.

This white sauce is perfect for vegetables, and it can be spiced up for chicken, seafood, or anything else you are cooking. It is also the base of many creamy soups with the addition of more milk and/or broth. However, this recipe keeps the calories and sodium down to a minimum.

The addition of sautéed mushrooms produces an excellent sauce for chicken. Adding chopped pieces of cooked chicken gives you chicken á la king. Two tablespoons of Parmesan cheese will also transform this sauce, giving it extra flavor. *Yield: 1 cup (4 ¼-cup servings)*

Ingredients

2 tablespoons low-fat margarine

2 shallots, peeled and minced

2 tablespoons all-purpose flour

1 cup warm low-fat milk

¹/₂ teaspoon salt

¹/₄ teaspoon Worcestershire sauce

¹/₂ teaspoon ground white pepper

Optional: ¹/₈ teaspoon ground nutmeg; 1 teaspoon chopped chives; 1 teaspoon sweet paprika; 1 hard-boiled egg, chopped; 1 teaspoon curry powder; or 1 teaspoon prepared Dijon-style mustard

Calories 85, **Fat** (g) 5, **Carbohydrates** (g) 8, **Protein** (g) 3, **Fiber** (g) 0, **Saturated Fat** (g) 1, **Cholesterol** (mg) 3, **Sodium** (mg) 3, **Carb Choice** ½, **ADA Exchange** ½ starch, 1 fat

Basic White Sauce

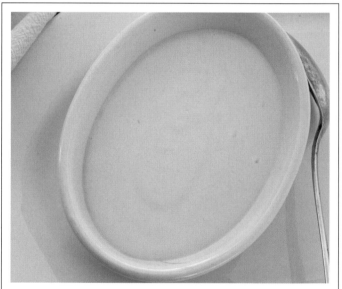

- Heat margarine in a saucepan over medium heat. Stir in minced shallot and cook until softened.

- Whisk in flour and cook, stirring until well blended with the margarine, about 3 minutes.

- Stir in warm milk, adding it slowly and making sure it blends, or you will have lumps.

- Mix in salt, Worcestershire sauce, and pepper. Reduce heat to low, and stir until very smooth and creamy. Add any of the optional ingredients you desire; serve.

Turning your white sauce brown: You can completely change this sauce by substituting 1 cup beef broth for the milk. Brown sauce is superb with all sorts of meats, especially if you mix it into the drippings in the bottom of the pan after you've roasted or broiled a piece of beef. Sautéing 1 cup of mushrooms with the shallots is also a nice addition to the sauce.

Varying the flavor: Vary the flavor by adding 1 tablespoon dry red wine to the brown sauce. Adding ½ cup roasted, peeled, and chopped chestnuts will make the brown sauce perfect for roast beef or venison. To make a spicy, hot sauce, simply sauté 1 chopped jalapeño pepper along with the shallots.

Making a Smooth Sauce

Turning a White Sauce into a Brown Sauce

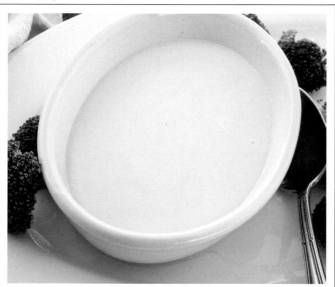

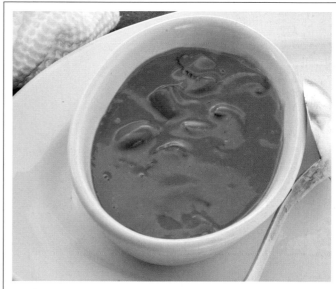

- If you don't sauté the flour prior to adding the milk, you will end up with a lumpy sauce and a raw flavor.

- If you add cold as opposed to warm milk to the sauce, you will get lumps.

- When adding lemon juice, do so just before serving, or the sauce will curdle (i.e., separate).

- Curdled sauce is lumpy, with an undesirable separation between the whey of the milk and the oils.

- When you are sautéing the shallots in the melted margarine, add ½ cup chopped mushrooms, to turn this into a brown sauce.

- Substitute warm beef broth for the warm milk. Follow the recipe as directed.

- Serve with roast beef or steak, or add to stew.

- You may also flavor the sauce with ¼ cup red wine.

MANGO SALSA
The perfect recipe for the cook who wants easy and elegant results

Mangos have been cultivated for 6,000 years in Southeast Asia and India. They are in the same family as cashew nuts, pistachios, and poison ivy.

There are 40 varieties of mangos, varying in skin color from red to yellow to purple. Mexico is the world's largest exporter of mangos. They are the most eaten fruit in the world, growing generously in warm climates.

Mangos are an excellent source of vitamins A and C. Because they are, like most fruit, high in sugar, a little bit of salsa goes a long way. So serve it by the tablespoon or as a dip. A little bit mixed with low-fat mayonnaise is wonderfully tasty. *Yield: 1 cup, depending on size of mango (serve by the tablespoon or as a dip, 24 servings)*

Ingredients

1 tablespoon olive oil

¼ cup finely chopped onion

2 serrano (for extra hot) or jalapeño (for just plain hot) chili peppers, seeded and finely chopped, more or less to taste

1 clove garlic, peeled and chopped

1 teaspoon ground cumin

1 inch peeled gingerroot, minced

Salt to taste

Pinch of Splenda

2 large or 3 medium mangos, peeled and chopped

Juice of 1 lime

2 tablespoons fresh cilantro, minced

Mango Salsa

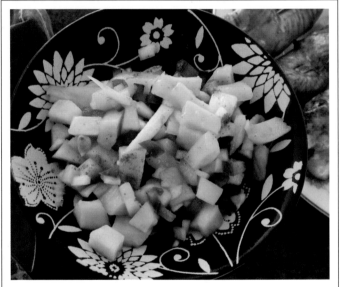

- Heat oil in a sauté pan over medium-high heat. Stir in onion, chilies, garlic, cumin, and ginger.

- Cook, stirring often, until vegetables soften. Place in a large bowl, and add the remaining ingredients.

- Cover and refrigerate for 30 to 60 minutes before serving.

Calories 111, **Fat** (g) 4, **Carbohydrates** (g) 21, **Protein** (g) 1, **Fiber** (g) 2, **Saturated Fat** (g) 1, **Cholesterol** (mg) 0, **Sodium** (mg) 4, **ADA Exchange** 1 fruit, 1 vegetable, 1 fat

Serving mango salsa: When you serve mango salsa as a dip for cold cooked shrimp, your guests will ask you for the recipe, and you may have to make a second batch. Mango salsa is also great spooned over cold chicken, lamb, or lobster. The lobster can be served hot or cold, and the mango salsa can replace butter or mayonnaise as a dipping sauce. Mix it with mayonnaise and add it to turkey salad. Fruit goes amazingly well with seafood, poultry, and meats. Most people serve cranberry relish with turkey and applesauce with pork, but fruit salsas are much spicier. Serve mango salsa on the side.

Removing a Pit from a Mango

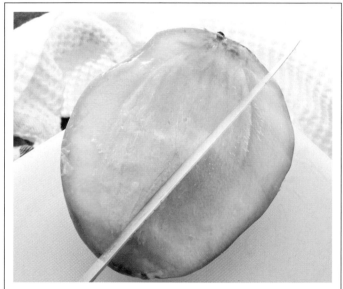

- To remove a pit from a mango, first cut the mango in half and twist it to release one side.

- Bang the side of the knife with the sharp edge down into the pit.

- Pull the pit out of the mango by retracting the knife from the fruit.

- Do not peel the mango. If you aren't going to use it immediately, sprinkle the fruit with lime juice to keep it fresh.

Dicing the Mango

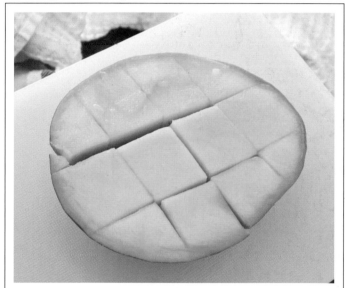

- Make ¼-inch cuts crosswise through the unpeeled mango. Do not pierce the skin.

- Make cuts lengthwise without piercing the skin. You will see the mango has been divided into a dice.

- Using a spoon, scrape the fruit from the skin and into a bowl.

- Be sure to use the mango soon after slicing to ensure freshness.

BAKED PEARS WITH CLOVES

A classic dessert is lightened up with low-fat vanilla yogurt

Baked pears are a fall natural, served warm and well spiced; you will find everyone loves them.

You can use almost any kind of pear for this recipe; 240 varieties are grown worldwide. If they are thin skinned, such as Bartlett, you don't even have to peel them; however, they will absorb more wine if you do.

Garnishing the pears with toasted walnuts or pecans right on top of the vanilla frozen yogurt is also wonderful. Although traditional recipes call for a sweet wine, this one does not. The sweetness comes from the pears and a bit of Splenda.

The pears can be baked for just a little while or al dente, or for long enough for the wine to become syrupy. *Yield: 4 servings*

Ingredients

4 ripe pears, peeled, cut into halves, cored

24 whole cloves

1/2 cup dry red wine

1/4 cup water

2 teaspoons Splenda

1 teaspoon orange zest

Topping: sugar-free vanilla frozen yogurt

Calories 143, **Fat** (g) 2, **Carbohydrates** (g) 31, **Protein** (g) 1, **Fiber** (g) 8, **Saturated Fat** (g) 0, **Cholesterol** (mg) 0, **Sodium** (mg) 19, **Carb Choices** 2, **ADA Exchange** 2 fruit

Baked Pears with Cloves

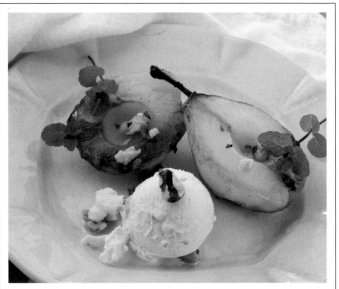

- Preheat oven to 350°F. Use nonstick spray on a baking dish that will hold the pears without overlapping.

- Arrange pears cut side down in the dish. Stud each pear half with 3 whole cloves. Add the liquids. Sprinkle pears with Splenda and orange zest.

- Bake until pears are soft, about 20 minutes, basting from time to time.

- Turn pears, cut side up, onto serving dishes. Add spoonfuls of frozen yogurt. Drizzle sauce over the tops of the pears.

Simple and sensational: You can whip up this appetizer in no time. It's especially refreshing in late summer, when pears are first available. Cut 2 small ripe pears in half, and remove the cores. In a small bowl, combine 4 tablespoons ricotta cheese with 1 tablespoon chopped pistachio nuts. Spread this mixture onto the cut sides of the pears, and garnish with a few extra whole pistachio nuts.

Make a quick pear sauce to serve with chops. Core 2 firm but ripe pears; cut pears into ½-inch slices. Add pears to pan in which you cooked chops. Sprinkle pear slices with 1 tablespoon Splenda and ½ teaspoon crushed dried rosemary. Cook over medium-low heat 3 minutes, stirring often. Pour ½ cup apple juice into pan; return pork to pan; simmer 5 minutes.

How to Core a Pear

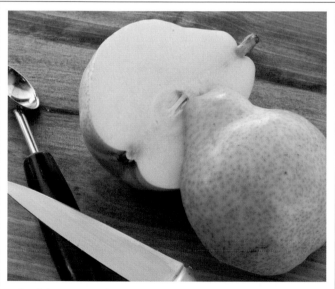

- Peel the pear, and cut it in half lengthwise.

- Using a paring knife, remove the stem and cut around the core.

- With a melon ball scoop, twist a circle around the core, and gently remove it.

- If your melon ball scoop doesn't go all the way around the core, the pear is likely to break.

Know When a Pear Is Ripe

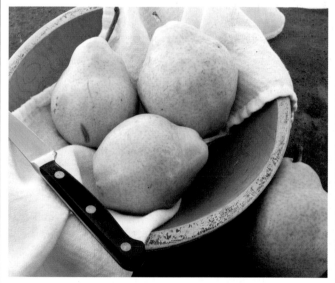

- To find out whether a pear is ripe, first sniff it. The pear should have a rich, fruity aroma.

- Then, using a paring knife, snip off a tiny bit of the fruit, right next to the stem.

- If it's hard and difficult to get the knife in, the pear is not ripe.

- If the knife slides into the stem end easily and drips juice, it's ripe and ready to eat.

DESSERTS

WATERMELON SORBET

Picture-pretty berries add to the high nutritional value of this dessert

Watermelon is an extremely low-calorie food. One cup contains only 46 calories that are packed with phytochemicals that are thought to boost your resistance to certain types of cancer.

The addition of the lemon juice and zest adds tang to this sorbet. The rule of thumb for "power" fruits and vegetables is that the deeper and more intense their color, the more nutritious and valuable they are for cancer prevention.

Watermelon not only boosts your "health esteem," it is also practically a multivitamin unto itself, containing excellent levels of vitamins A (important for optimal eye health), B6 (used to manufacture brain chemicals that help us cope with anxiety), and C (which helps bolster the immune system). *Yield: 4 servings*

KNACK DIABETES COOKBOOK

Ingredients

2 cups watermelon, seeds removed, no white or green part

Juice and zest of $1/2$ lemon

3 teaspoons Splenda, or to taste

Pinch of salt

Dash of Tabasco sauce (optional)

1 cup fresh blueberries, washed and picked over

4 fresh mint leaves

Calories 45, **Fat** (g) 0, **Carbohydrates** (g) 12, **Protein** (g) 1, **Fiber** (g) 1, **Saturated Fat** (g) 0, **Cholesterol** (mg) 0, **Sodium** (mg) 79, **Carb Choice** 1, **ADA Exchange** 1 fruit

Watermelon Sorbet

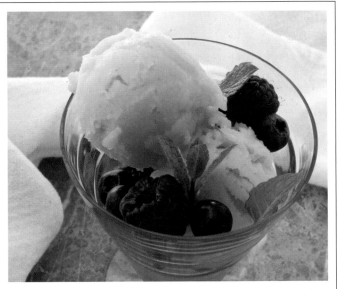

- Place the first four ingredients and Tabasco sauce, if desired, in a blender.

- Whirl until pureed; the mixture will expand a bit when blended. Stop the blender from time to time to scrape down the sides.

- Place in an ice cream maker and freeze according to the manufacturer's directions.

- Serve garnished with fresh berries and a mint leaf.

Watermelon sorbet: Watermelon sorbet can take on a whole new flavor by the addition of 2 blanched peaches to the recipe. Simply add the seeded peaches to the watermelon while you are blending it. Make dessert smoothies with watermelon sorbet. Just add 1 cup of sugar-free lemon or lime yogurt and blend.

One cup of fresh raspberries also makes a good addition to the sorbet as you freeze it. The whole berries freeze into icy nuggets that are very tasty and do not require any added sugar. Your sorbet will be a different color if you use yellow or golden watermelon instead of the red/rosy variety. For a complete change of pace, make sorbet using honeydew or cantaloupe melon. The same quantities of melon and the same directions work just fine.

No Ice Cream Freezer?

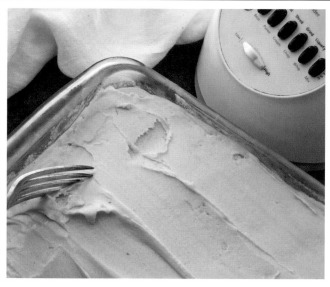

- Place the sorbet in a freezer container or a baking pan normally used for brownies.

- Place in the freezer. When it begins to freeze, whisk the sorbet with a fork.

- When the sorbet is quite stiff, break it up and put it back into the blender.

- Return to the freezer. When stiff, place in a plastic container and keep frozen until ready to serve.

Distinguishing Sorbet, Sherbet, and Ice Cream

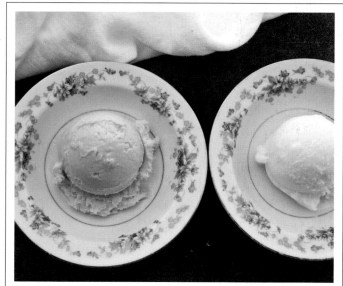

- Sorbet is basically an ice. Sherbet is an ice that also contains milk.

- Sherbet comes in almost as many flavors as sorbet.

- If you make your own sorbet (or sherbet), you have fewer calories, and you control the amount of sugar and the type of fruit.

- Ice cream is a sorbet base with the addition of heavy cream and sometimes eggs, as in ice cream custard.

DESSERTS

PEACH FLAN

The naturally sweet taste of summer is now available year-round

Flan is an incredibly simple dessert. It is equally good in the summer as it is in the winter. Very popular in France, Spain, and Italy, this dish uses various seasonal fruits.

Flan can also be made as a very rich custard, such as crème caramel renversé. This classic and super-rich dessert is made with lots of whole eggs and cream. Butter is caramelized on the bottom of a ring-form mold. When the custard has cooked, it's turned over to make it renversé.

This recipe has just fruit and more egg whites than yolks. The same creamy, satiny effect is achieved with very few calories, and the sweetness from the peaches and Splenda is quite enough. *Yield: 6 servings*

Ingredients

6 large ripe peaches, blanched for skin removal, pitted, and sliced

Juice of ¹/₂ lemon

1 cup low-fat milk

¹/₄ cup Splenda for baking

¹/₃ cup all-purpose flour

¹/₃ cup whole-wheat flour

3 egg whites

2 whole eggs

2 teaspoons pure vanilla extract

¹/₂ teaspoon salt

Calories 167, **Fat** (g) 3, **Carbohydrates** (g) 28, **Protein** (g) 9, **Fiber** (g) 3, **Saturated Fat** (g) 1, **Cholesterol** (mg) 72, **Sodium** (mg) 75, **Carb Choices** 2, **ADA Exchange** 1 starch, 1 fruit, 1 very lean meat

Peach Flan

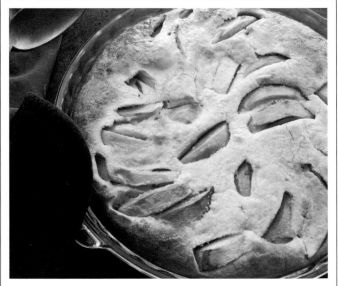

- Preheat oven to 350°F. Sprinkle sliced peaches with lemon juice. Toss.

- Place remaining ingredients in a blender, pulsing after each addition.

- Set a stovetop burner on medium. Spray glass pie pan with nonstick spray.

- Add enough batter to make a thin coat on bottom of pan.

- Place pan on the burner 2 to 3 minutes to set batter.

- Remove from heat; place peaches on top of set batter. Pour in remaining batter; bake 1 hour.

Peach substitutions: Flan can be made with apples, pears, berries—just about any fruit you like and whatever's in season. For apple flan, peel, core, and slice 4 large apples. Sprinkle with ½ teaspoon cinnamon, and proceed as you would with peaches. Have fun by mixing fruit when you make flan. Try adding ½ cup dried cranberries to the apple flan, and 1 cup fresh or frozen blueberries to the peach flan. You can also try plums and nectarines in the flan. If you leave the skins on thin-skinned fruit, you will add to the fiber content of the flan. This is especially true of plums and nectarines, as well as certain varieties of pears. Make use of whatever comes in season.

Blanching Peaches

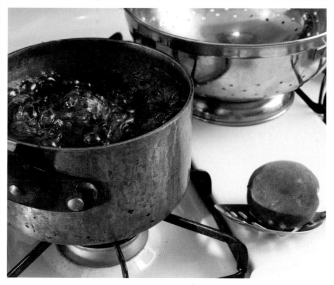

- Many fruits require blanching to remove their skins. Blanching is far more efficient than peeling, which removes a great deal of fruit along with the skin.

- To blanch, start with a pot of boiling water. Ease one piece of fruit at a time into the pot; return to a boil before adding more.

- After a minute or so, remove the fruit with a slotted spoon, and place in a colander. Let cool.

- Using a paring knife, slip the skin from the fruit, and place the blanched fruit in a bowl.

Acid and Oxidization

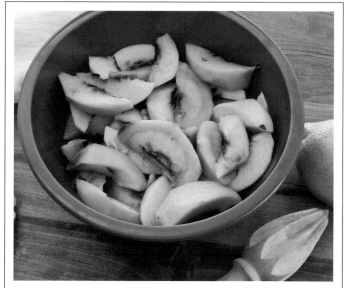

- Apples, bananas, potatoes, peaches, and pears are some of the foods that will turn brown when exposed to oxygen.

- The brown is not harmful but can be unsightly.

- To prevent this, add vinegar or citrus juice to the item that will brown.

- In the case of peaches, apples, or bananas, simply toss them with some lemon, orange, or lime juice. Vinegar is better for potatoes.

DESSERTS

221

MERINGUE TART WITH FRUIT

An Old World dessert is brought up-to-date with American flair

Originally called "Pavlova cake," this dessert was named after the famous Russian ballerina. There is controversy over the exact origin of the recipe. Some food historians say it was created in Australia; others claim it came from Europe.

To make the crust even more interesting, fold ¼ cup ground nuts into the stiff egg whites. Another good addition is fresh lemon or orange zest.

Meringue tarts are rather spectacular. However, there is one warning: If you are in a humid climate, make the crust at the last minute. Humidity in the air or from boiling or steaming food in the kitchen will soak into the tart crust, making it gummy. *Yield: 8 servings*

Ingredients

For the tart shell:

5 egg whites

1 tablespoon all-purpose flour

$^1/_2$ teaspoon white vinegar

2 tablespoons Splenda (for baking)

For the filling:

1 banana, peeled and sliced

$^1/_2$ cup whipping cream, whipped, or low-calorie whipped topping

1 pint strawberries, washed, stemmed, and sliced

1 tablespoon Splenda

Calories 85, **Fat** (g) 3, **Carbohydrates** (g) 11, **Protein** (g) 4, **Fiber** (g) 2, **Saturated Fat** (g) 2, **Cholesterol** (mg) 11, **Sodium** (mg) 50, **ADA Exchange** 1 fruit, ½ lean meat

Meringue Tart with Fruit

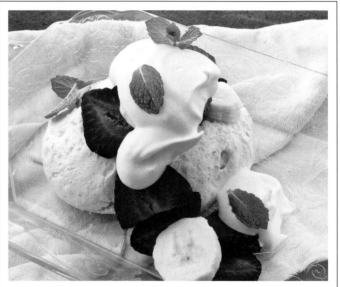

- Preheat oven to 250°F. Whip egg whites until foamy; add flour and keep beating. Add vinegar and Splenda; whip until high, stiff peaks form.

- Using a pastry bag, form 8 meringue shells of equal size on a baking sheet. Bake 60 to 90 minutes, or until shells dry out. Turn oven off; open the door slightly. Leave shells in oven.

- When dry, place slices of banana on bottom of each. Cover with whipped cream and strawberries. Sprinkle with Splenda. Add more whipped cream in dollops on top. Decorate with reserved berries.

Separating Egg Whites

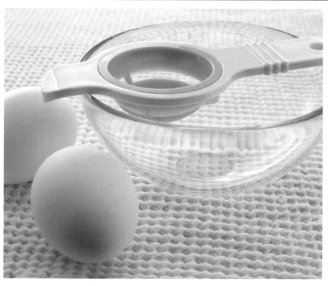

No Yolks, Grease, or Fat

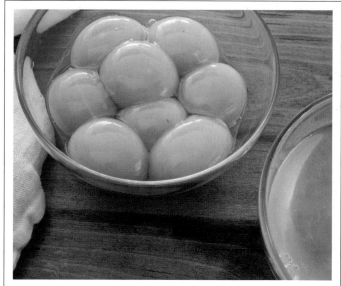

- There is a tool for separating yolks and whites. Place it over a cup or bowl, and break the egg over it. The yolk remains in the separator while the white slips through slits on sides.

- After the egg is split, tip it so that the yolk sits in the small end of the shell. Pour the egg white into a bowl. Slide the yolk into the other shell.

- Add the rest of the white to the bowl. Pour the yolk into the empty second bowl.

- Examine the egg white carefully to make sure there is no yolk in it.

- In order to whip eggs whites into stiff peaks, there cannot be even a tiny speck of yolk in the whites.

- The beaters must be grease-free and immaculately clean, or the eggs will not whip into peaks.

- The bowl in which you whip the eggs must also be totally clean and grease-free.

- If there is even a bit of yolk, grease, or fat on any part of the equipment, the eggs will foam slightly but not get stiff.

DESSERTS

WALNUT-STUFFED BAKED APPLES
Old-fashioned baked apples are as delicious as apple pie and less fattening

Almost every variety of apple is suitable for baking. You can use the Macintosh, a sweet/tart apple, or a much more tart apple, such as the Greening or Granny Smith, but there are hundreds of others from which to choose.

Some apples, such as green ones, are higher in sugar than others. All apples—especially when eaten with the skin on,

as in this recipe—are high in fiber. They are also high in phytochemicals, which are cancer preventatives, and they promote regularity, as any high-fiber food does. Hence the old saying, "An apple a day keeps the doctor away."

This recipes provides a healthful alternative to your standard apple pie dessert. *Yield: 4 servings*

Ingredients

4 teaspoons finely chopped walnuts

4 teaspoons Splenda brown sugar

1 teaspoon cinnamon

4 large apples

2 teaspoons low-fat margarine

1 cup all-natural apple cider or apple juice

4 tablespoons sugar-free vanilla frozen yogurt or sugar-free ice cream

Calories 199, **Fat** (g) 5, **Carbohydrates** (g) 41, **Protein** (g) 3, **Fiber** (g) 6, **Saturated Fat** (g) 1, **Cholesterol** (mg) 1, **Sodium** (mg) 30, **Carb Choices** 3, **ADA Exchange** 3 fruit, 1 fat

Walnut-Stuffed Baked Apples

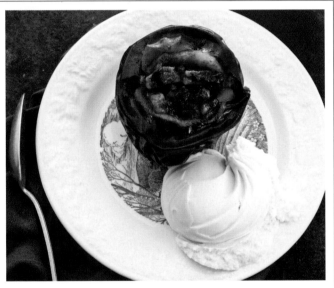

- Preheat oven to 350°F. Prepare baking dish with nonstick spray. Mix walnuts, Splenda, and cinnamon in bowl.

- Core apples. Stuff nut mixture into apples.

- Arrange apples in dish close together so that they prop

each other up and don't fall over. Dot tops of apples with low-fat margarine. Pour cider over tops.

- Bake 25 minutes. Don't let cider burn off; add more cider or water if necessary. Serve with 1 tablespoon frozen yogurt or ice cream.

Baked stuffed apples cut in half: Baked stuffed apples don't always have to be cored with a vertical hole going down the center. Try simply cutting the apple in half from top to bottom, and scooping the core out with a grapefruit spoon or melon ball scoop. Place apple skin-side down in a baking dish. Mound the entire half with 1 heaping tablespoon mixed chopped nuts, raisins, Splenda, and the spices in the recipe. Sprinkle with 1 tablespoonful bread crumbs. Moisten each apple with 1 tablespoon apple juice or cider and 1 teaspoon low-calorie margarine. Bake until apple halves are softened and topping is golden brown. Alternatively, mound chopped nuts, pecans, almonds, or walnuts on apples. Sprinkle chopped nuts with fresh orange zest and moisten with orange juice.

Grilled Fruit

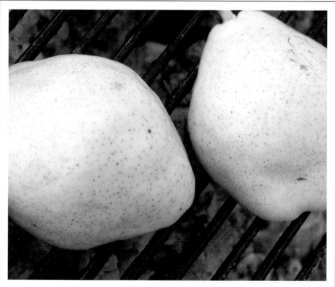

- Many types of fruit are excellent when cooked on a charcoal or gas grill as opposed to being baked in the oven.

- When you grill a pear or peach, do not skin the fruit.

- Brush the fruit with lemon juice. You don't have to grill fruit for a long time, just until it's very hot.

- Because it's drier than baked fruit, grilled fruit needs to be dressed with a sauce, a bit of low-fat margarine, or a sweetened cheese, such as low-calorie cream cheese mixed with Splenda.

Macerated Fruit

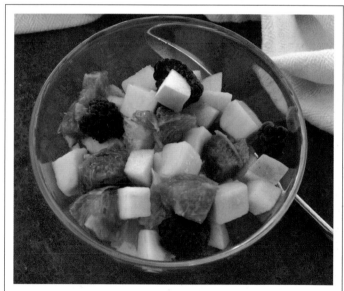

- Macerated fruit is basically fruit that's been "cooked" in ascorbic acid from citrus. This is an easy way to prepare a variety of fruit.

- Mix together 4 cups various seasonal fruits, such as bananas and pineapples, that have been peeled, pitted, and cut into pieces.

- Add ½ cup orange juice, 1 teaspoon curry powder, and Splenda to taste. You can also use a liqueur, but this will add sugar and calories.

- Toss to coat well. Let "cook" in the refrigerator for 1 to 2 hours, then serve.

DESSERTS

225

PUMPKIN SOUFFLÉ

Pumpkin is an excellent source of vitamin A that takes naturally to many kinds of spices

The great American pumpkin is an early sign of the autumn harvest, of full moons and Halloween. The best pumpkins to eat are called "sugar" pumpkins, but all are edible. The smaller, round ones are just sweeter than the big oval ones.

Millions of tons of pumpkin meat go to waste every year as holiday decor and in the making of jack o' lanterns. Many pumpkins become fodder for animals, and millions are processed for pies.

Canned pumpkin is sold plain, unseasoned, and unsweetened, or tricked out with sugar and spices. It's best to use your own sweetener, salt, and spice so that you can control the amounts of each. *Yield: 6 servings*

Ingredients

³/₄ cup canned pumpkin puree

2 tablespoons Splenda brown sugar

1 teaspoon cinnamon

¹/₈ teaspoon nutmeg

¹/₄ teaspoon ground cloves

¹/₂ teaspoon salt

1 tablespoon orange juice

5 egg whites

2 tablespoons sugar-free vanilla-flavored frozen yogurt

Calories 53, **Fat** (g) 0, **Carbohydrates** (g) 8, **Protein** (g) 4, **Fiber** (g) 2, **Saturated Fat** (g) 0, **Cholesterol** (mg) 1, **Sodium** (mg) 67, **Carb Choice** ½, **ADA Exchange** ½ starch

Pumpkin Soufflé

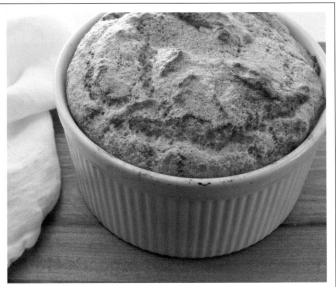

- Preheat oven to 375°F. Prepare a 1-quart soufflé dish with nonstick spray.

- Whisk puree, Splenda, cinnamon, nutmeg, cloves, salt, and orange juice in a saucepan, and warm over low heat.

- Beat egg whites until stiff peaks form. Fold the pumpkin mixture into the whites; pour into the soufflé dish.

- Bake 20 to 25 minutes. Spoon onto dishes, top each serving with 2 tablespoons frozen yogurt, and serve immediately.

Nuts and soufflés—perfect contrasts: Swirling ½ cup toasted, ground pecans into the pumpkin mixture before adding the egg whites will add a different flavor and texture. Walnuts and almonds are very good, too. Simply grind them in a food processor after toasting them on top of the stove or under the broiler. The nuts add fiber to the dish, which lessens the effects of the naturally sweet pumpkin pulp.

Fruits to add to pumpkin soufflé: Dried cranberries, golden raisins, or diced dried apricots are both sweet and flavorful. A little bit of dried fruit goes a long way. Soak ½ cup dried cranberries or other fruits in 1 cup hot water. When they plump, drain and add them to your pumpkin soufflé. For a change, substitute sugar-free applesauce for the pumpkin, but use the same spices as in this recipe.

Using Canned Pumpkin

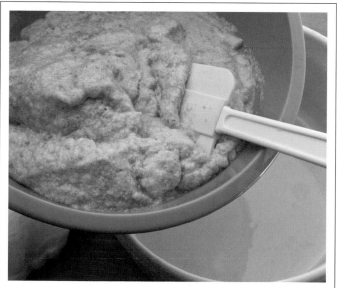

Using Butternut Squash

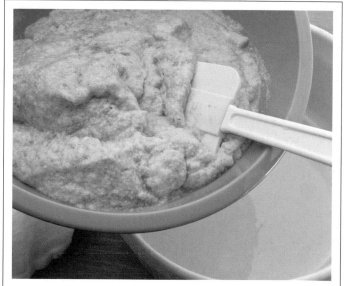

- Canned pumpkin is a great time-saver. Some supermarkets sell skinned and cut-up fresh pumpkin.

- You can boil prepared fresh pumpkin, or microwave it 8 to 10 minutes or until soft. Then puree it in your blender.

- Do not buy canned pumpkin that's been sweetened and spiced. It's loaded with sugar and overly seasoned.

- Butternut squash is in the same family as the pumpkin. Both are varieties of winter squash.

- Butternut squash is available frozen year-round.

- You may have to cook frozen butternut squash down, reducing it, as it is usually quite watery.

- When you've reduced a 9-ounce package to ¾ cup, add the spices and Splenda. Then proceed with the recipe.

DESSERTS

WEB SITES & TV SHOWS
General information for people with diabetes

Healthy Cooking TV Shows

Get Fresh with Sara Snow
The Discovery Network
www.discovery.com

Healthy Appetite with Ellie Krieger
The Food Network
www.foodnetwork.com

Healthy Cooking with Dr. Kosta and Dave
PBS
www.pbs.com

Living Fresh with Sara Snow
The Discovery Network
www.discovery.com

Healthy Cooking Web Sites

All Recipes
www.allrecipes.com

Cooking Light
www.cookinglight.com

DLife
www.dlife.com

Eating Well
www.eatingwell.com

Epicurious
www.epicurious.com

Foodfit
www.foodfit.com

Healthy Cooking Recipes
www.healthycookingrecipes.com

Lowfat Lifestyle
www.lowfatlifestyle.com

Mayo Clinic
www.mayoclinic.org

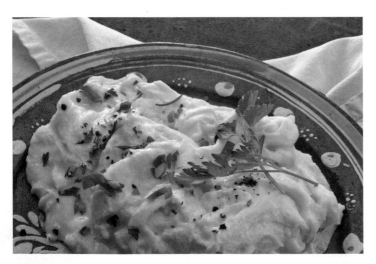

Organizations

American Diabetes Association
www.diabetes.org

American Dietetic Association
www.eatright.org

Children with Diabetes
www.childrenwithdiabetes.com

Directory of Diabetes Organizations
http://diabetes.niddk.nih.gov/resources/organizations.htm

International Diabetes Federation
www.idf.org

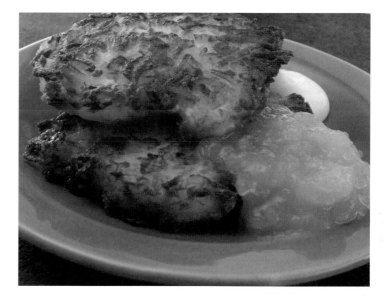

Jewish Diabetes
www.jewishdiabetes.org

Juvenile Diabetes Research Foundation International
www.jdrf.org

National Diabetes Educational Program
www.ndep.nih.gov

National Institute of Diabetes and Digestive and Kidney Diseases (NIDDK)
www.niddk.nih.gov

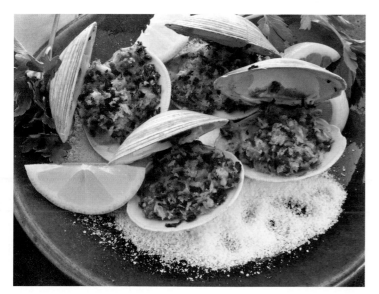

MAGAZINES & OTHER RESOURCES

Magazines

Cooking Light
www.cookinglight.com

Diabetic Cooking
www.diabeticcooking.com

Diabetic Living
www.diabeticlivingonline.com

Eating Well
www.eatingwell.com

Everyday Food
www.everydayfood.com

Heart Healthy Living
www.hearthealthyonline.com

Taste of Home
www.tasteofhome.com

Newsletters

American Diabetes Association
www.diabetes.org

Diabetes in Control
www.diabetesincontrol.com

Juvenile Diabetes Research Foundation International
www.jdrf.org

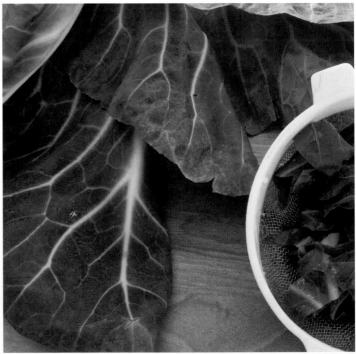

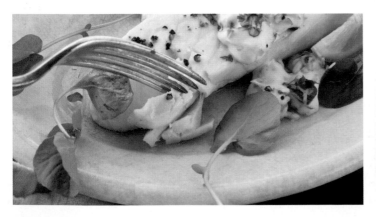

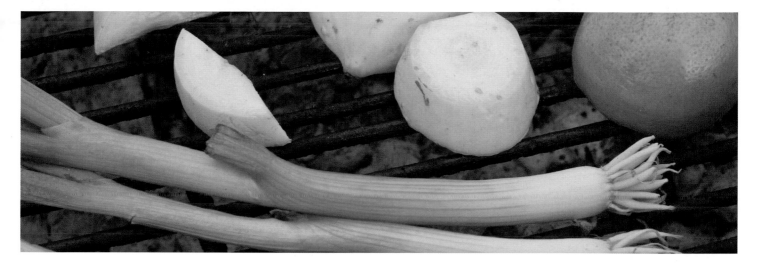

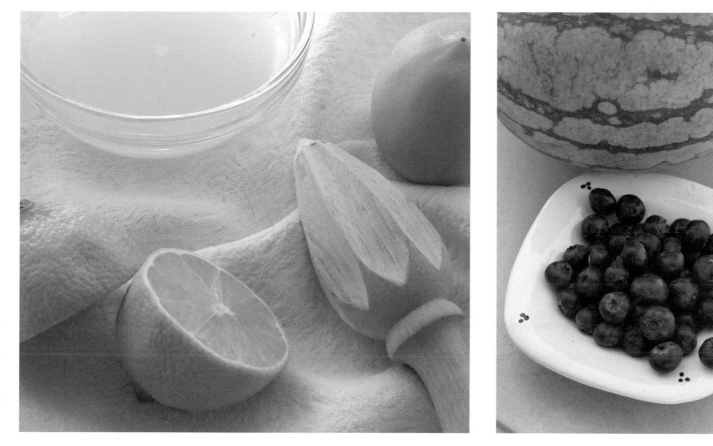

EQUIPMENT RESOURCES

Find equipment through these resources to stock your kitchen

Catalogs for Cooking Equipment

Brylane Home
- Lots of kitchen equipment, including specialty tools, utensils, and dishware

Solutions
- Lots of new equipment and tools to make cooking quick and easy

Williams-Sonoma
- Top-of-the-line equipment, along with cookbooks and many appliances, tools, and accessories

Sur la Table
- Catalog offers lots of kitchen equipment, along with dishes, serving utensils, and flatware

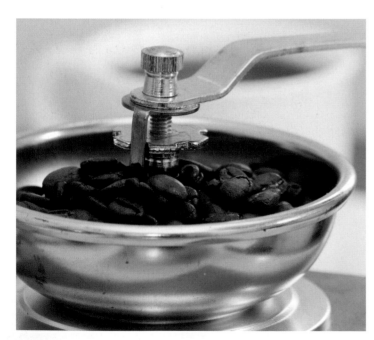

Kitchen Cooking Equipment

Crock-Pot.com
- Web site for Rival slow cookers, this site offers customer service, replacement parts, and recipes.

Cooking.com
- Kitchen fixtures, large appliances, cutlery, cookbooks, and tools can be found at this site.

ChefsResource.com
- Cutlery, flatware, gadgets, tools, knives, and brands like Cuisinart are featured.

KitchenManualsOnline.com
- Web site offers contact information for dozens of slow cooker manufacturers.

Grilling Equipment Manufacturers

Weber Grills
www.weber.com
- Weber grills are classic. This manufacturer of the original kettle grill also makes sophisticated gas grills and a wide variety of tools.

Coleman Grills
www.coleman.com
- The Coleman Company makes equipment for outdoor living; not just grills, but camping equipment, too.

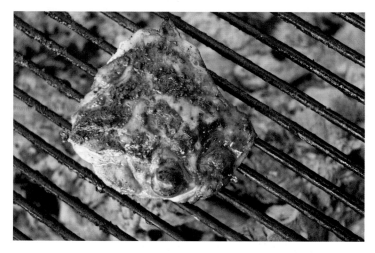

Big Green Egg
www.biggreenegg.com
- The Big Green Egg is a heavy duty cast-iron grill and smoker that will literally last a lifetime. And uses much less fuel than traditional grills.

Jenn Air
www.jennair.com
- Jenn Air specializes in large, well-equipped gas grills. It also offers equipment and tools to complement the grills.

Fiesta Grills
www.fiestagasgrills.com
- Fiesta offers four lines of grills, ranging from simple gas grills to complete built-in kitchens.

Holland Grills
www.hollandgrill.com
- Holland grills are designed to prevent flare-ups because a drip pan is permanently installed between the food and the burners.

Viking Grills
www.vikingrange.com
- These premium, high-end grills are all meant to be built into a custom outdoor kitchen.

GrillSearch
www.grillsearch.com
- This website lists just about all of the grill manufacturers in the world. Links to websites and equipment information.

Hearth, Patio & Barbecue Association
www.hpba.org
- This association offers product information, news about products and recalls, recipes, and service locators.

Soup Equipment Web Sites

Crock-Pot.com
- The Web site for Rival slow cookers, this site offers customer service, replacement parts, and recipes.

Cooking.com
- Information on kitchen fixtures, large appliances, cutlery, cookbooks, and tools can be found at this site.

ChefsResource.com
- Cutlery, flatware, gadgets, tools, knives, and brands like Cuisinart are featured.

KitchenManualsOnline.com
- Web site offers contact information for dozens of slow cooker manufacturers.

FIND INGREDIENTS

RESOURCES

Farmers' Markets

FarmersMarketLA.com
www.farmersmarketla.com
- Los Angeles Farmer's Market website; the original farmer's market.

National Directory of Farmer's Markets
www.farmersmarket.com
- Site has index of U.S. Farmer's Markets listed by state.

Farmer's Market Search
apps.ams.usda.gov/FarmersMarkets
- USDA site lets you search for a farmer's market by state, city, county, and zip code, as well as methods of payment.

Organic Foods

Cedarlane
www.cedarlanefoods.com

Eden Organic
www.edenfoods.com

Horizon Organic
www.horizonorganic.com

National Grocer's Association
www.nationalgrocers.org

Purity Foods
www.purityfoods.com

Small Planet Foods
www.smallplanetfoods.com

Trader Joe's
www.traderjoes.com

Whole Foods Market
www.wholefoodsmarket.com

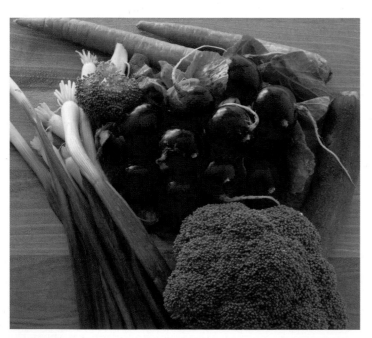

METRIC CONVERSION TABLES

Approximate U.S. Metric Equivalents

Liquid Ingredients

U.S. MEASURES	METRIC	U.S. MEASURES	METRIC
¼ TSP.	1.23 ML	2 TBSP.	29.57 ML
½ TSP.	2.36 ML	3 TBSP.	44.36 ML
¾ TSP.	3.70 ML	¼ CUP	59.15 ML
1 TSP.	4.93 ML	½ CUP	118.30 ML
1¼ TSP.	6.16 ML	1 CUP	236.59 ML
1½ TSP.	7.39 ML	2 CUPS OR 1 PT.	473.18 ML
1¾ TSP.	8.63 ML	3 CUPS	709.77 ML
2 TSP.	9.86 ML	4 CUPS OR 1 QT.	946.36 ML
1 TBSP.	14.79 ML	4 QTS. OR 1 GAL.	3.79 L

Dry Ingredients

U.S. MEASURES		METRIC	U.S. MEASURES	METRIC
17⅗ OZ.	1 LIVRE	500 G	2 OZ.	60 (56.6) G
16 OZ.	1 LB.	454 G	1¾ OZ.	50 G
8⅞ OZ.		250 G	1 OZ.	30 (28.3) G
5¼ OZ.		150 G	⅞ OZ.	25 G
4½ OZ.		125 G	¾ OZ.	21 (21.3) G
4 OZ.		115 (113.2) G	½ OZ.	15 (14.2) G
3½ OZ.		100 G	¼ OZ.	7 (7.1) G
3 OZ.		85 (84.9) G	⅛ OZ.	3½ (3.5) G
2⅘ OZ.		80 G	¹⁄₁₆ OZ.	2 (1.8) G

HOTLINES & MANUFACTURERS

Find help with cooking problems and equipment manufacturers

Hotlines

USDA Meat and Poultry Hotline
1-800-535-4555
- Year-round line offers information about food safety, answers consumer questions about meat preparation.

Empire Kosher Poultry Hotline
1-800-367-4734
- Year-round hotline answers questions about poultry.

Butterball Turkey Holiday Line
1-800-323-4848
- Hotline available year-round; for answers to questions about turkey cooking and preparation.

Reynolds Turkey Tips
1-800-745-4000
- Year-round hotline answers consumer questions about turkey preparation; free recipes.

Perdue
1-800-473-7383
- Year-round hotline helps with cooking questions, especially for poultry products.

Manufacturers of Equipment

Rival
www.rivalproducts.com
- Manufacturer of the original Crock-Pot, with product information, recipes, and an on-line store.

All-Clad
www.all-clad.com
- One of the first manufacturers to make metal inserts for the slow cooker.

KitchenAid
www.kitchenaid.com
- Lots of high quality appliances offered, from refrigerators and stoves to slow cookers.

General Electric
www.geappliances.com
- Outfit your entire kitchen with General Electric appliances. Online service and customer support.

Cuisinart
www.cuisinart.com
- Complete kitchen outfitter, from ranges to stock pots.

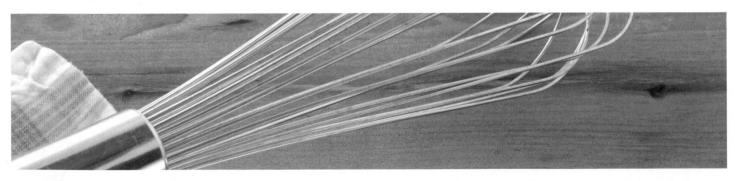

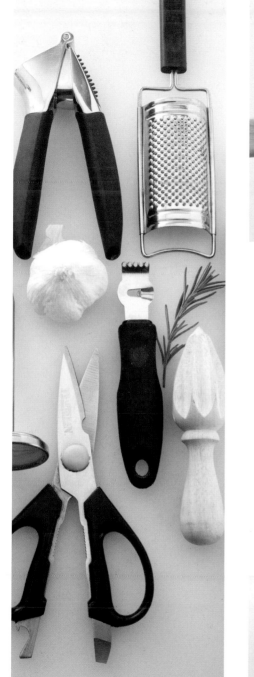

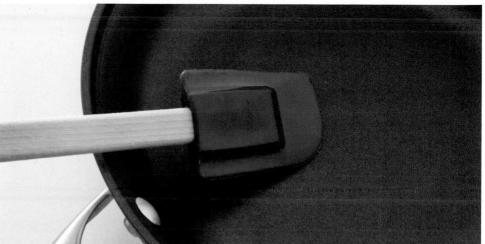

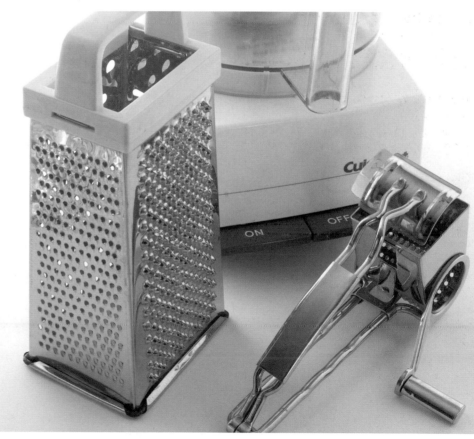

237

GLOSSARY
The language of cooking

Baste: To cover food with a sauce or marinade while cooking.

Beat: To manipulate food with a spoon, mixer, or whisk to combine.

Blanch: To briefly cook, primarily vegetables or fruits, to remove skin or fix color.

Bread: To coat meat with crumbs or crushed crackers before baking or frying.

Broil: To quickly cook food close to the heat source.

Broth: Liquid extracted from meats and vegetables, used as the basis for most soups.

Brown: Cooking step that caramelizes food and adds color and flavor before cooking.

Caramelize: A chemical reaction catalyzed by heat which combines sugars and proteins to form complex flavors and colors in grilled food.

Charcoal: Real charcoal is made by burning solid wood in a controlled atmosphere without carbon; it becomes almost pure carbon.

Chill: To refrigerate a soup or place it in an ice-water bath to rapidly cool.

Chop: To cut food into small pieces using a chef's knife or a food processor.

Coat: To cover food in another ingredient, as to coat chicken breasts with bread crumbs.

Deglaze: To add a liquid to a pan used to sauté meat; this removes drippings and brown bits to create a sauce.

Dice: To cut food into small, even portions, usually about ¼-inch square.

Flake: To break into small pieces; canned meats are usually flaked.

Fold: To combine two soft or liquid mixtures together using an over-and-under method of mixing.

Grate: A grater or microplane is used To remove small pieces or shreds of skin or food with a grater or microplane.

Grill: To cook over coals or charcoal or over high heat.

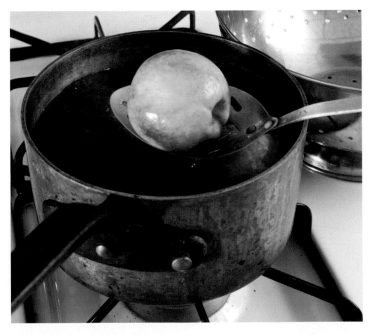

Marinade: A mixture of an acidlike citrus, oil, and seasonings used to flavor meat, fruits, and vegetables before grilling.

Marinate: To stand meats or vegetables in a mixture of an acid and oil to add flavor and tenderize.

Melt: To turn a solid into a liquid by the addition of heat.

Pan-fry: To cook quickly in a shallow pan in a small amount of fat over relatively high heat.

Shred: To use a grater, mandoline, or food processor to create small strips of food.

Simmer: A state of liquid cooking, where the liquid is just below boil.

Skewer: As a noun, a sharp metal or wooden stick threaded with food. As a verb, to place food on a skewer to make kabobs.

Slow cooker: An appliance that cooks food by surrounding it with low, steady heat.

Soup: A mixture of solids and liquids served hot or cold, as a main dish or part of a multicourse meal.

Steam: To cook food by immersing it in steam or setting it over boiling liquid.

Toss: To combine food using two spoons or a spoon and a fork until mixed.

Whisk: As a noun, a tool made of varying loops of steel; as a verb, a method of combining ingredients until smooth and blended.

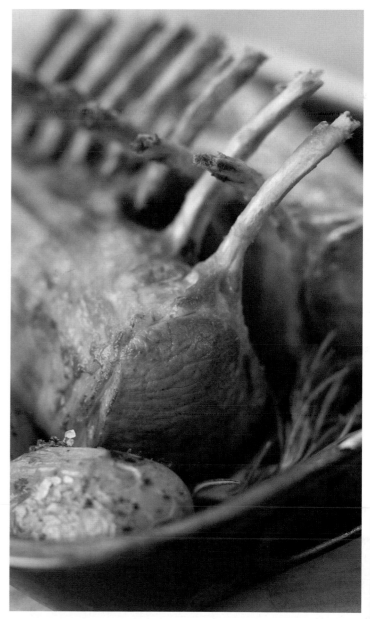

INDEX

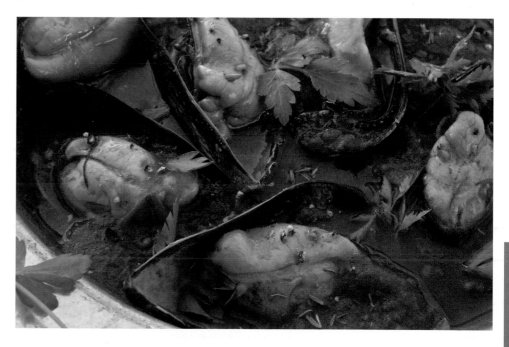

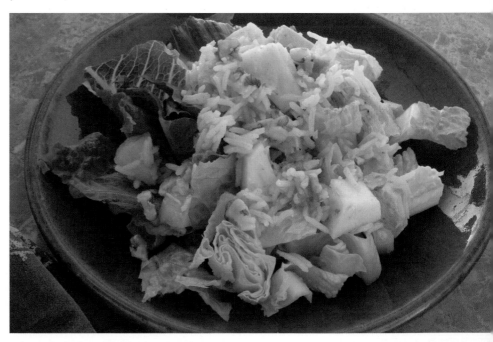